REFORMING HEALTI

What's the evidence?

Ian Greener, Barbara E. Harrins
Russell Mannion a

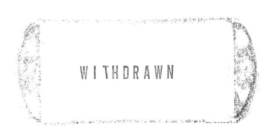

WITHDRAWN

First published in Great Britain in 2014 by

Policy Press
University of Bristol
6th Floor
Howard House
Queen's Avenue
Clifton
Bristol BS8 1SD
UK
Tel +44 (0)117 331 5020
Fax +44 (0)117 331 5367
e-mail pp-info@bristol.ac.uk
www.policypress.co.uk

North American office:
Policy Press
c/o The University of Chicago Press
1427 East 60th Street
Chicago, IL 60637, USA
t: +1 773 702 7700
f: +1 773-702-9756
e:sales@press.uchicago.edu
www.press.uchicago.edu

British Library Cataloguing in Publication Data
A catalogue record for this book is available from the British Library

Library of Congress Cataloging-in-Publication Data
A catalog record for this book has been requested

ISBN 978 1 44730 710 5 paperback
ISBN 978 1 44730 711 2 hardcover

Cover design by Robin Hawes
Front cover: istock
Printed and bound in Great Britain by CMP, Poole
Policy Press uses environmentally responsible print partners

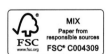

Contents

List of tables

Acknowledgements

The authors would like to thank the NIHR HS&DR (National Institute for Health Research Health Services and Delivery Research) funding programme for providing the resources on which this book was based: Grant number 08/1808/245: A realistic review of clinico-managerial relationships in the NHS: 1991–2010.

Barbara also wishes to thank Kate, Lesley and Roger Clark, and Steve, Trish and Sam Harrington.

ONE

Introduction

> I used to pore over the latest offerings from various highly reputable academic or scholarly quarters, and find nothing of any real practical help. (Tony Blair, cited in Powell, 2011)

During the 2000s there was a great deal of rhetoric about evidence-based policy and evidence-based policy-making (Davies et al, 2000; Perkins et al, 2010). However, policy and policy-making often appear to be rather more based on the existing ideas (or even prejudices or ideologies) of those in positions of power rather than on research evidence. And there are several reasons for this.

Policy-makers may believe they already know what needs to be done, and so do not need to examine what research says. Equally, those in positions of power may find research inaccessible in terms of its place of publication, or that it is written in dense, academic language they find difficult to understand. They may also find research to be too equivocal, too concerned with trying to consider both sides of a problem than coming to a conclusion or solution that they can get on with turning into a workable policy. Policy-makers may also have strong views about what needs to be done by government, regardless of what researchers are telling them, often seeming to put their own political goals ahead of research, and their ideology ahead of evidence.

When looking back at NHS reorganisations, it does seems to be the case that since the 1980s policy-makers have been unable to resist changing organisational structures, not even waiting to see if the last changes they attempted to put into place had worked or hadn't. Secretaries of State for Health have sometimes seemed as if they are intent on leaving their own impression on the NHS organisation without considering whether what they are planning to change has any real chance of working.

From the perspective of academics and researchers, on the other hand, policy-makers and politicians often appear to have short attention spans and do not want to engage with the complexities of the area they are trying to change. Politicians can sometimes look as if they have decided what needs to be done without looking at lessons from the past or from other countries.

As a result, the dialogue between politicians, policy-makers and academics engaged in research can be a series of miscommunications and misunderstandings. Academics can appear to be engaged in spurious debates over arcane points that they spend their lives writing about in unclear language, rarely saying what actually needs to be done, and policy-makers trying to repeatedly reorganise public services based on little other than their belief that doing so will somehow make things better. There is now, for example, a great deal of evidence on the difficulties of achieving successful structural healthcare reorganisation, but this basic insight doesn't seem to deter policy-makers from engaging in yet another ... healthcare reorganisation.

In the last 20 years, things have, in some respects at least, improved on both sides. Policy-makers have made greater use of academics and academic research, with respected social policy writers such as Chris Ham and Julian Le Grand being brought in to advise ministers in key social policy areas. Academics have tried to write for non-academic audiences, becoming aware that they must create an 'impact' outside, as well as inside, the 'academy'. But there still appear to be relatively few examples of the gap between government and the academy leading to productive policy-making and the kind of close relationship between policy and research that we might hope for.

This book synthesises research on health service reorganisation in the UK, but particularly in England, over the last 30 years, to try and explain not only what seems to have worked best, but also how we might incorporate those findings into present and future health service reform. To 'reform' means to change things for the better. As we will see, however, too often service reorganisation has either made things worse, or failed to achieve the desired goals while ignoring research evidence in the process. We need to do better. Academic research can be made more accessible, and clear findings presented in a form that might lead to health services being improved.

The evidence considered in this book is mainly concerned with work conducted in the English National Health Service (NHS), but its general lessons go well beyond England; it considers research from other countries in the UK that require us to pause and reflect whether the pro-market approach taken in England really is the best way forward. The book aims to make a contribution to understanding the principles on which healthcare reorganisation can work better more generally, as well as considering the nature and type of evidence on which such judgements can be made. Not every academic will agree with what follows, but we hope that this book can be the beginning of a conversation about how health services can be improved, as well as contribute towards the debate about how evidence from research can be used to that end. If we succeed in these goals, we will have made a useful contribution.

Reviewing research on healthcare reform

> I do not propose to go into the pros and cons of these different NHS organisational structures as it is tedious beyond belief and, in the end, all such reorganisations have proved remarkably unsuccessful at causing anything to change aside from letterheads and job titles. (Taylor, 2013, p 86)

Roger Taylor, founder of the Dr Foster website (see www.drfosterhealth. co.uk) that provides data on the performance of health services, provides us with a salutary reminder of the difficulty of reviewing research on healthcare reorganisation. Although we must discuss reorganisations at some level of detail, we must also acknowledge that doing so can result in what looks like arcane, acronym-based discussions that appear to have little relevance to anyone not directly interested in the detail of NHS organisational structures. To avoid this, we need a rigorous method that brings existing research together to produce robust findings on which policy-makers can act, and which may even be generalisable to other public services. We need a method for considering existing studies and trying to synthesise what they have to say.

The standard way of reviewing existing research is through what is often called a 'systematic review'. This involves conducting a literature search, often using computerised databases, then considering whether the studies found fit within the scope of the review being conducted. The systematic approach then assesses whether each study is of sufficient quality to be included. Finally, when the research that has met both the relevance and quality criteria has been identified, those in charge of the synthesis combine the research findings in various ways, giving extra weight to the research that is regarded as being the highest quality. This 'systematic' approach is based on practice in clinical research, and is often regarded as the 'gold standard' approach to evidence synthesis.

However, when research is about organisations and people (which attempts to reorganise healthcare undoubtedly are), the systematic approach outlined above simply does not work. First, it assumes that findings are not tied to particular contexts, assuming that the mark of good research is generalisable and that it can be applied in whichever context it is needed. The systematic approach pays little or no attention to the particular time, place and people it researches – it treats healthcare reorganisation as something that has the same impact on everyone, with everyone having the same problems to deal with. The particular organisational context is often a crucial factor in whether an attempt at reorganisation will be a success and deliver the desired improvements. A moment's reflection surely shows that health services in the most deprived areas of the country will need to work in a different way from those in the most affluent areas.

This isn't to say that health services in different areas have nothing in common, but we do need a way of trying to take account of context which is neither so particular that we can learn nothing from it for other organisations, or so abstracted from context (which is what tends to happen in the systematic approach) that it applies to no one.

Second, the systematic approach assumes that the organisation or organisations being reorganised are effectively closed systems. Closed systems get their name from being insulated from their environment. This is useful as it focuses our attention on factors that are inside the organisations that we are studying, and allows us to try and isolate the specific factors that are causing improvements or problems to occur. In clinical research we can put in place controls and experimental interventions to try and measure the efficacy of the treatments we are researching (with varying degrees of success), but in organisations there is always a wide range of different external factors that are likely to interfere with our organisations at any one time. One example in healthcare is the 'inverse care law' advanced by Tudor Hart (1971), which suggests that those in the most deprived areas often have the worst access to good health services, as clinicians often don't want to live in such areas. Not only that, but people in the most deprived areas also seem the most reluctant to seek care in the first place. If people are struggling to find work or good housing and are living on low incomes, then there is a clear environmental effect on health services even before we take into account the problems of recruiting and retaining good clinicians in such areas. This all leads to a series of complex problems that are beyond the direct control of the clinicians and managers working within them. Open systems – those affected and shaped by their environment – mean that we have to be extremely careful in making claims that particular changes have led to specific results – it is almost always less straightforward and more complicated than that.

Finally, there may well be gold standards of what counts as good evidence in clinical research (although in some quarters this is a matter of dispute), but in organisational and policy research these standards do not exist to anything like the same extent. Different academic disciplines have their own standards of what counts as good research, and it may well even be that what appear to be poorly conducted studies have something important to contribute to our understanding of healthcare reorganisation, especially as the field is often so fast-moving that it is difficult to conduct the high-quality, long-term research we might ideally want.

Realist review

This book attempts to tackle the challenges outlined above by taking what has become known as a 'realist review' approach (Pawson et al, 2005; Pawson, 2006). Such a review still searches existing research to assess what it says, but does not make the same judgements about the quality of research that should be included or excluded in the review. Instead, the realist review approach takes a more theory-driven approach – with 'theory' meant not in an abstract way, but in the sense of 'there's nothing so practical as a good theory'.

The first step in realist review is to search for and assemble research that examines a given healthcare reorganisation – in common with the systematic approach. Beyond that, however, it works in a different way. Rather than applying quality-based criteria to include or exclude which studies should be included, a realist review attempts to find the best theory of what seems to have happened. It does this by separating the context of the research as much as possible from the particular changes that the reorganisation introduced (the mechanisms), and from their outcomes or results. By doing so, we can begin to build theories not only of what worked (as measured by the outcomes), but also in what contexts and for whom. We can look for patterns of context, mechanism and outcomes, and try and generate insights based on these patterns that help us better understand the complex, open systems that make up modern healthcare.

Central to the realist review approach is the need to be able to generate 'programme theories' – by which we 'surface' the theories which appear to underlie policy proposals – and to be able to examine their success in a range of different contexts and settings. We can then evaluate reorganisations in a contextually sensitive way, as well as coming up with comparisons where similar ideas for reorganisation appear to have been tried in very different settings. This means, for example, we can compare the use of performance management in hospitals and GP practices to get a better sense of how well it has worked in each setting, to better inform both in the future. We therefore need to try and find similar reorganisation mechanisms with sufficient in common in order to be able to compare their use in different contexts. This requires us to take a creative and reflexive approach to research review, rather than using a simple checklist of quality criteria and trying to use a fixed approach for turning hundreds of studies into a single final synthesis. It is therefore possible that different researchers would produce a different review of the research considered in the writing of this book, and the research report on which it is based. This is not to dismiss what follows as merely 'subjective', but instead to acknowledge that any synthesis or evaluation of research involves decisions about what is most important. In the words of Pawson (2013, p 86), realist review requires 'organised scepticism' as the 'superintending force' of the approach, as an evaluation or review necessarily has to make such 'unavoidable' judgements. Here we have chosen to foreground those judgements rather than to try and hide them away through an opaque research method.

As such, the realist review approach aims to generate theory that can be abstracted and applied to different contexts. We can learn about performance management in the NHS, but also generate findings that can be applied in different contexts as well, so long as we are sensitive to those new contexts and reflexively ask whether the findings we have generated can be applied there too.

Establishing the context within which programme theories are being introduced is a challenge within realist review. Working out which factors are important analytically, and which we can leave out of our account, again requires careful judgement and thought. However, it seems possible to make a few generic points, derived particularly from the work of Margaret Archer, another researcher who has placed realism at the heart of her work (see, for example, Archer, 1995). Archer suggests that we need to explore continuity (which she calls 'morphostasis') and change ('morphogenesis'), exploring the effects of context on how human agents understand and act, as to do so is to recognise that different contexts have properties that necessarily inhibit or support people in their everyday lives. Archer suggests that we need to especially consider what she calls 'structural' conditionings – about how groups interact with one another – and what their sources of power might be, and 'cultural' conditionings – which ideas are important in any context in terms of how they help actors understand their world – and whether those ideas are broadly complementary or conflicting with one another. Both structure and culture do not determine how human agents behave, but they do make some courses of action either easier or more difficult than others.

Following Archer, we explore the political (broadly structural) and ideational (broadly cultural) context in each time period explored in the book, to establish what influence it is likely to have on any attempts at organisational change. We need to consider the political context into which a programme theory is being introduced – especially in terms of the relationships between key groups such as politicians, doctors, nurses and patient groups. In any period we need to know which groups appear to be most important in terms of establishing the context for reorganisation, and how relations between them are configured. Who appears to be in control? Who has the power of veto?

As well as needing to consider the political context, we also need to consider the world of ideas. According to what principles are organisations being run in each period? Are doctors running things according to a professionalised view of the world, or are managers challenging them through the introduction of budgets and performance management systems? How is the NHS being held to account?

Considering the political and ideational context in each period gives us a basis for considering the context into which programme theories are being introduced, as well as obtaining an initial sense of their likely success – if doctors are in charge, then we might reasonably infer that reorganisations based on managerial ideas are unlikely to be successful.

The final aim of realist review is not definitive evidence that one intervention works better than another in all contexts, because such a goal is unachievable. Instead it aims at producing an explanation that 'brings to light the reasoning to be gone through in making decision' (Pawson, 2006, p 169).

Reviewing health reorganisation, 1990–2013

It is not possible to capture and explore the introduction and effects of every single policy in the health service context since 1990, as the 2000s, in particular, have been a time of policy and reorganisation hyperactivity in which it often seemed as if every week brought forth new announcements and initiatives.

What we do here is examine health service policy change and reorganisation around the two broad approaches that policy-makers described as taking place in the 2000s – those that were designed to exert greater command and control, and those that were an attempt to generate local dynamic improvement – and to examine example policies or reorganisations under each of these headings. Command and control changes included the considerable extension of performance management initiatives that dominated the early part of the 2000s (and which never really went away during that period). Local dynamic reorganisation, on the other hand, was based on the idea of (re) introducing a market and increasing patient and public involvement in healthcare, and dominated policy-making in the second half of the 2000s (although it was also partially present before then). Neither of these headings is pure or absolute – performance management, as we will see, can be introduced to allow considerable local discretion in terms of implementation, and the introduction of a market for care, although meant to lead to local organisations competing and generating a local dynamism, requires a great deal of central government intervention to put it in place. But the two types are sufficiently distinct to be analytically separable, and considering them one at a time can help illuminate our understanding of the dynamics of public reorganisation.

Dividing different reorganisation into these two categories also allows us to generate findings that have the potential to be generalisable. By grouping attempts at reorganisation this way it allows us to compare, for example, different types of performance management. Performance management has acquired a bad reputation in healthcare due not only to research showing substantial difficulties in relation to the way its measures have been 'gamed' in hospitals, but also because it has been singled out as a central feature of the 'corporate' approach that led to a failure of care at Mid Staffordshire Hospital in the report of the second Francis Inquiry into those events (see Francis, 2013). But an institution such as the NHS, dependent on public funds and accountable to Parliament for these, does require some kind of central control, and, we argue, it is possible to learn lessons about how performance management can work better from its use in general practice (GP) surgeries – through the Quality and Outcomes Framework (QOF). By comparing attempts at performance management in hospitals with the QOF in GP surgeries we can generate a theory of when performance management works, and when it does not, that can help inform policy and practice, as well as explaining how it can be made to work better even in contexts, such as hospitals, where it appears to have been more problematic. This means that the theories generated here allow us to generalise from one context (such as GP surgeries) to different contexts (such as hospitals), as well as offering valuable, theory-driven lessons for other healthcare systems.

What follows here is not an attempt to summarise all the research that examines the NHS since 1990, but an attempt to come up with the strongest and most robust explanations we can manage of what does and does not appear to work in healthcare reorganisation, grounded in practical theories that can inform future such reorganisations, not only in the UK, but in other countries as well. We can then also reflect on the nature of the realist review process, and what it means for the kinds of evidence that we need in order to evaluate healthcare reorganisations better.

Structure of the book

The structure of the book is as follows. We begin by outlining the organisational form of the NHS in 1990, the date with which our review of NHS reorganisation begins. This starting date gives us the 30 most recent years of evidence to draw upon, but also because research evidence up to 1990 has already been well summarised by the work of Harrison, Hunter and Pollitt (see, for example, Harrison, 1988; Harrison et al, 1990, 1992; Pollitt et al, 1991b). The year 1990 therefore provides a good date to start reviewing healthcare reorganisation, as well as being the time at which the first internal market for care was introduced into the NHS, so representing the beginning of several attempts to reorganise healthcare on pro-market and pro-competition principles. As NHS organisation, especially post-2005, takes healthcare markets to be its central concern, evidence around them is an important part of the book's contribution.

Having set the context for healthcare in 1990, we then outline the many attempts to reorganise healthcare between 1990 and 2010, taking the reader through the introduction of the first internal market, the election of the 'New Labour' government in 1997, the NHS Plan in 2000, the raft of reorganisations that took place during the 2000s, and the controversial coalition government reorganisation post-2010. To explore these changes in more detail, we then categorise reorganisations under two main headings, as suggested above. The first type of reorganisation attempted to achieve greater central control through the use of performance management and the greater standardisation of care in both hospitals and GP surgeries ('central control'), and the second type, although it was introduced through government policy (and so was very much centrally imposed), sought to achieve improvement through 'local dynamism', through the reintroduction of a healthcare market and by giving a stronger voice to patients through the reorganisation and patient and public forums.

There are certainly other ways of thinking about health policy in the 2000s, but we would argue that this account represents a good way of being able to compare different reorganisation attempts (by comparing 'central control' mechanisms, for example), and of developing theories that can help inform future debates about healthcare reorganisation.

The book concludes, first, by considering the prospects for success of the coalition government's NHS reorganisation, based on the research evidence from the rest of the book, and second, by suggesting alternative principles that might have a better chance of working.

Finally, it is important to stress that although this book is about healthcare, it is not an example of what has become known as health service research. Instead, it is an explanation of the relationship between social policy and public management that attempts to examine the case of the NHS since 1990 to consider what we can learn about how to reorganise public services to improve them, and how we can use existing research to that end. This is an important distinction – the NHS here is the case study that we use to explore the dynamics of public reorganisation, and although the book, we would argue, makes a contribution to how healthcare might be improved, it is not about healthcare in the broadest sense. It is about how the UK government has attempted to reorganise the NHS, examining research on that topic since 1990 with a view to drawing lessons about public service reorganisation more generally that can apply both to the NHS and to other services in the UK and elsewhere.

It is time to make a start. What was the NHS like in 1990, and how have policy-makers attempted to reorganise healthcare since then?

TWO

The NHS in 1990

Introduction

The aim of this chapter is to provide the context for the rest of the book, exploring the NHS in 1990 in terms of its organisational structure and dynamics at that time. In an institution like the NHS, where understanding history is important to get a sense of why particular structures were put in place or what kinds of relationships exist between policy-makers and staff, this necessarily involves going back before 1990. However, we attempt to include only the elements of NHS history that are most relevant to understanding the material in the rest of the book.

The chapter proceeds by presenting the background to health organisation and policy in 1990 to provide a starting point for the account of subsequent reorganisations, exploring in more depth attempts at reorganisation during the 1980s (especially the Griffiths management reforms and the *Working for patients* internal market) in order to construct the 'shared version' of health politics in 1990s which provides the starting point, and context, for the book's analysis.

Background

The central organisational relationship in health policy and politics in the first decades of the NHS was that which existed between the state (broadly speaking, the government of the day) and the medical profession. Klein (1990) captures the relationship in characteristically vivid terms as being a 'double bed' of mutual dependence, with the medical profession dependent on the state which was effectively the monopoly employer of their services (outside of a very small private sector), and the state, at the same time, dependent on the medical profession to both run the NHS, and to ration its care within the resources available. Although the relationship was one of dependence, that did not mean that conflict could not occur or even become public (as it certainly did during negotiations over medical contracts in the 1960s and during industrial disputes in the 1970s), but it did mean that both the state and the medical profession had little alternative but to try and work with one another to make the best of the situation.

The period 1948–81 was, in retrospect, one of remarkable continuity and relative calm in respect of NHS organisation and policy. During this time there was only one attempt at significant NHS reorganisation (in 1974, which was the product of 10 years' debate over the best way to proceed), and the 1979 Royal Commission examining the NHS was broadly supportive of the NHS at that time. By the early 1980s the NHS was still remarkably similar to the organisation created by the NHS Act of 1946.

In terms of its day-to-day running, those working for the NHS had a great deal of autonomy from central government. The right of clinicians to practice largely free from managerial control ('clinical freedom') was a central principle around which the NHS was organised (Klein, 1990), and Harrison and Pollitt (1994) suggest that the service provided by the NHS as a whole in the early 1980s was the aggregate outcome of individual doctors' decisions in choosing which patients to treat and when. The autonomy given to the medical profession in running health services meant that there was little or no managerial oversight of their activities, and doctors were portrayed as operating within their own 'fiefdoms' of control (Giaimo, 1995, p 358).

From the 1960s through to the 1980s, however, increased concern was being expressed by groups representing patients (including those involved in disability rights) that health services seemed to be organised rather more around the needs of professionals than those of their patients (Southon and Braithwaite, 1998). The academic literature in the meantime became more critical and less accepting of professionals in society, suggesting that groups such as doctors were often more interested in preserving and building their own power and status, or in engaging in interprofessional 'tribal' rivalries, than in trying to achieve the broader societal good that their representative bodies tended to espouse (Abbott, 1988; Baggott, 1995).

NHS management, or to use the contemporary term, 'administration', was, in comparison to the US or developed European economies, under-resourced, and carried little status or financial reward. Healthcare managers were more often regarded as facilitators for doctors than as leaders, or as carrying any authority themselves, and large areas of the NHS, especially GP surgeries, were almost entirely free from managerial oversight and control. As such, in the early 1980s, NHS management was in many ways representative of the 'old public administration' style of governance (Hood, 1991), with doctors effectively running local health services through their own hierarchy, and the managers or administrators who were in place there to support them in their work. There was a paucity of local management information, and little political will or authority to attempt to exert increased control over doctors.

Things were, however, beginning to change. The NHS was in the hands of a government that was generally sceptical about the benefits of public services, and regarded the medical profession less as a professional grouping and more as a closed-shop trade union that was blocking change (Harrison, 1988; Klein, 1990). The reorganisation of the NHS in the 1970s demonstrated that the medical profession expected a seat at the table in order to discuss the content of any significant change (Klein, 1979), and that a government-led challenge to clinical autonomy would trigger significant opposition from the doctors who could be expected to mount campaigns against the government that would risk unpopularity with the public, which opinion polls suggested trusted doctors a great deal more than trusted politicians. It is against this background that the Conservative governments' attempts at NHS reorganisation during the 1980s need to be considered.

Reorganising healthcare in the 1980s

The NHS management inquiry or Griffiths report

Despite the remarkable continuities in health policy up to the 1980s, that decade began a period of increasingly frequent reorganisation. Early in their first term in office, the Conservatives removed a tier of organisation put in place by the 1974 reorganisation, and experimented with a more decentralised approach to organising healthcare (Klein, 2006). By 1983 the government wanted to go further. The Thatcher government asked Roy Griffiths (Deputy Chairman of Sainsbury's) to investigate the way the health service was run. Griffiths' report (DHSS, 1983) was presented as a 23-page letter to the Secretary of State for Health, Norman Fowler, rather than a detailed report – in marked contrast with the volumes of evidence presented by the recent Royal Commission (Merrison, 1979).

Griffiths claimed that the NHS suffered from a lack of individual management accountability, was reactive to problems rather than strategic and proactive, that there was a lack of focus on performance and almost no evaluation of its services, and that managers displayed a lack of concern for their customers' views of the services they were receiving. Griffiths recommended that a Supervisory Board should be created which would work under and report to the Secretary of State, taking on all responsibilities for NHS management, and including non-NHS managers among its membership. Under the Health Services Supervisory Board, general manager posts would be created in regional and district health authorities so that individual accountability was established in those organisations, but with those managers being allowed discretion in how they achieved the goals they set. Instead of having a permanent post, general managers would be appointed on five-year fixed-term contracts. Reviews of services were to be carried out more widely at unit level with the aim of reducing costs without impairing services, and clinicians (especially doctors, who Griffiths regarded as the 'natural managers' of the NHS) were to be more involved in local management, and given workload-related budgets for which they would be held responsible. Finally, NHS services were to pay more attention to patients, community groups and their viewpoints through closer working with the community health councils set up in 1974, supplemented by market research so that they knew what their customers wanted.

So the *NHS management inquiry* presented the problems of the NHS as being due to a lack of effective management, and given this problematisation, it is perhaps unsurprising that the solution was for the NHS to become more business-like, with clearer lines of accountability, doctors taking greater responsibility for the service they provided, and for patients to be treated more like customers with needs that it was the responsibility of managers to meet. On top of this, however, there was the more radical idea that health services might be allowed to differ from one area to the next, as local managers were given greater autonomy to meet local needs so long as the managers were also held accountable for those services. This was a challenge to the idea of the NHS attempting to provide a single standard of service across the country, even if this was always more an aspiration given the very significant differences in service provision and effectiveness that persisted from one area to another (Powell, 1997).

The government largely accepted Griffiths' managerial proposals, but without allowing managers the discretion or authority to reconfigure their local services differently. Even without greater localism, the Griffiths' proposals were radical in that they tried to change the dynamics of health services so that managers moved away from the facilitative roles they had held in the past, towards a more proactive and strategic role instead, a move from consensus management to a general manager-led approach. But with this came the need to challenge the autonomy held by doctors who were used to running health services largely without managerial involvement.

However, it was not clear that general managers held the authority or power to meet the challenges of their new roles. On the ground, the reality of being an NHS manager in the 1980s was to be overwhelmingly concerned with financial problems and the need to find efficiency savings. The 1980s was a time when rising unemployment put considerable pressure on government finances, and budget rises for the NHS were kept to a minimum.

Faced by competing tensions between national initiatives and local needs, and the difficulties of getting clinicians to change practices and to be more accountable, it is perhaps unsurprising that there seems to be little evidence of general managers attempting to put in place radical change. If the Griffiths reorganisation was an attempt to introduce a more managerialist approach, or to encourage greater diversity and localism in health services, then it is hard to see that it achieved either goal.

Other changes during the 1980s

In addition to attempting to meet the challenge of the Griffiths report, a number of other changes were made to the NHS during the 1980s that went with the grain of the new more 'business-like' approach to organising healthcare.

First, the government put in place competitive tendering for domestic and catering services. This meant that private companies could now compete to provide their services inside an ostensibly public organisation. Whereas before domestic and catering services were another functional area within a hospital, staffed by full-time NHS employees, they were now often franchises of local or national cleaning or catering firms, even if they ended up employing the same staff who had worked in the hospital before (and often at a reduced rate of pay).

Second, as well as competitive tendering, the 1980s saw the introduction of performance measurement into the NHS (Pollitt, 1985), but again, it appeared to have little effect in either relationships between doctors and managers or in improving health services. It proved extremely difficult to come up with any consensus as to how the performance of healthcare organisations could be measured (Bloomfield, 1991), with doctors favouring systems that allowed them to be in control and which were geared to improving diagnosis, but which then had much less obvious managerial application (Harrison et al, 1992b).

Third, in 1984 the government issued restrictions on the right to prescribe, putting in place a 'limited list' of approved treatments which doctors could prescribe for patients in an attempt to standardise treatments, but also to try and reduce the costs of the ever-expanding NHS drugs bill by making sure the best value treatments were being prescribed through the use of generic medicines where possible rather than more expensive, branded alternatives. This was contentious in that it was a challenge to the medical profession as it directly interfered with the ability of doctors to prescribe medicine as they saw fit.

Fourth, the government began a 'more oblique approach' (Harrison and Pollitt, 1994) to challenging medical power in hospitals through a range of changes broadly badged as the 'resource management initiative' (Buxton and Packwood, 1991). As noted above, one of the changes suggested by the Griffiths report was to try and make doctors more accountable for their decisions through the use of devolved budgets. This accountability was one element of resource management (initially known as 'clinical budgeting'), but which also included attempts to increase the number of doctors in managerial roles, putting in place clinical management structures and the development of audit and quality improvement mechanisms.

The resource management initiative was implemented in three broad stages: first came the use of clinical budgets to try and encourage doctors to be more concerned with the costs of running their services; second came the more ambitious management budgets, which attempted to get managers and doctors to find savings and to improve efficiency within their services; and finally, resource management, which in addition brought into place mechanisms to attempt to get clinicians to audit one another and to find ways of improving the quality of the services that they offered.

The range of initiatives in the resource management programme still did not, however, lead to a significant challenge to clinical practice (Harrison et al, 1992b). Audit and clinical quality improvement processes were regarded as being 'off limits' for non-clinicians, so most managers found that they had few, if any, new levers to make clinicians more accountable for their decisions. The lack of reliable management information meant that clinician fiefdoms remained largely intact, and resource management systems developed in a state of 'organisational isolation' with little sharing either between different NHS organisations or even within the same ones (Harrison and Pollitt, 1994, p 90). The underlying information systems put in place to make resource management work were often chosen and implemented by clinicians rather than managers, leading to slow implementation, and appeared more geared to clinical than managerial interests (Brown, 1992).

As such, the changes originating from the *NHS management inquiry*, from the introduction of performance management and those coming from the resource management initiative in all its forms, appeared small in impact. Limited list prescribing was a challenge to doctors' right to prescribe as they saw fit, and contracting out of services gave general managers a tool in at least changing the way ancillary services were run, moving it onto a more contractual basis. In all, however, the introduction of general managers did not instigate a significant cultural change, with clinicians retaining their autonomy and power. Even the systems through which performance data were collected were largely under clinical control, as were audit and quality improvement processes.

Impact of changes during the 1980s on nurses and patients

The Griffiths management inquiry may have had the relationship between doctors and managers as its focus, but it also held the potential to have a significant impact on nursing. In response to concerns raised by nurses about other professionals holding budgets that were primarily concerned with nursing work, chief nursing officers were put onto management boards, and district health authorities were required to appoint a senior nurse in an advisory role.

The resource management initiative and quality management were, in contrast to the rather agnostic response they received from doctors, often embraced by nurses as a means of improving patient care. At the same time, however, nurses found their work monitored increasingly closely through the collection of management information, leaving them questioning why an initiative whose primary purpose was to challenge medical power appeared to being directed instead at them (Packwood et al, 1990; Buxton and Packwood, 1991). Nursing, in terms of its identity as a profession, appeared to be going through a crisis of confidence, made worse by a combination of recruitment shortages and the government introducing a national accreditation scheme in the face of opposition from the profession, and making the Royal College of Nursing appear as if it was struggling to defend its members. The less than robust professional status and representative power of nurses was in marked contrast to doctor representation groups such as the British Medical Association and Royal Colleges, which remained politically powerful and influential in representing their members. Project 2000 attempted to reform nursing education and raise its profile and status, but appeared to do little to revitalise the profession (Hart, 1994).

If nurses appeared to have gained little from the changes of the 1980s, what about patients? The *NHS management inquiry* was clear that the NHS needed to be more responsive to the need of patients, presenting them in customer-like roles in contrast to the more passive position of the grateful recipient of care patients had often occupied previously. In practice, however, little seemed to change. There was certainly an increased tendency for patients to question clinicians, and the deference offered to doctors in the early years of the NHS appeared to be declining, not least by the women's movement's critiques of practices such as episiotomy during childbirth (which appeared to be often done for the convenience of the doctor overseeing care rather than the mother), and by disability groups criticising the inflexibility and lack of care with which the NHS often treated those with both physical and mental disabilities (Clarke, 2004). There was certainly something in Griffiths' claim that patients increasingly regarded themselves as taking on more customer-type roles, wanting to be treated with care and respect and to be involved in care decisions made about them. Despite these changes, patient representative groups and the voice of the patient in health service design remained extremely weak, with the NHS remaining very much a producer-run service.

The road to *Working for patients* and the first internal market

The 1980s appeared to offer the lesson that it was remarkably difficult to change the inherited dynamics of the health service. Towards the end of the decade, frustrated by the lack of real change in the NHS, concerned about a rising drugs budget and an ageing population, and apparently goaded on a television programme about the government's record on the NHS, Prime Minister Thatcher announced that an NHS review was under way (Klein, 2006).

To begin with, the review appeared to be progressing slowly, with Secretary of State John Moore unwell and struggling to make the case for change in Parliament. Moore was replaced by the more robust Kenneth Clarke, who appeared to quickly come to the conclusion that moving NHS funding away from a general taxation-based system risked greater expense as it was an excellent way to keep a lid on costs (see also Lawson, 1991). Clarke's main innovation was in supporting the introduction of a purchaser–provider split – an idea that linked back to proposals from US economist Alain Enthoven, and which came from his visit to the UK earlier in the decade (Enthoven, 1985). Enthoven suggested that the NHS was 'riddled with perverse incentives' that resulted in inefficiencies, and which prevented clinicians and managers from improving services, even potentially punishing anyone who attempted to do so (Light, 1992). The solution, in Enthoven's eyes, was the introduction of market-like mechanisms into healthcare through the use of a 'quasi-market' that retained both the purchasing and provision of care in the public sector, but attempted to capture the dynamism and responsiveness of private sector competition.

The idea of using a market mechanism in reorganisation of the NHS resonated with a government that preferred private to public provision, and that had been asking health managers to become more 'business-like' for most of the 1980s. Interviews with the architects of the reorganisation, especially Kenneth Clarke, portray the reforms as offering continuity with earlier changes, but giving health managers a stronger authority because of the market-based challenges that they would now face (Ham, 2000).

In the White Paper that introduced the reorganisation, *Working for patients* (Secretary of State for Health, 1989), the government argued that reform was necessary because of rising demands for health services, the ever-expanding range of health services on offer, the wide variations in the cost and quality of treatment in the NHS, and its unacceptable waiting times. In common with the Griffiths report, the changes were presented as a means of decentralising control away from government to raise performance by giving increased autonomy to GPs and hospitals and to delegate responsibility:

> It [the government] is convinced that it can be done only by delegating responsibility as closely as possible to where health care is delivered to the patient – predominantly to the GP and the local hospital. (Secretary of State for Health, 1989, p 102)

Working for patients aimed to give patients a greater choice over the services available to them, extending the customer focus of the Griffiths reforms to a model where patients were also given a choice over the provision of their health services. At the same time, it suggested that the reorganisation would offer greater job satisfaction to those working within the NHS as a result of their increased ability to respond to local needs. Contracting out was to be extended, and consultants more involved in the management of their hospitals. There were objectives to increase the number of consultant posts, to get money to flow across organisational boundaries to better meet the needs of patients, and for large GP surgeries to be able to apply to become budget-holders in their own right so they would be able to purchase a defined range of services direct from hospitals. Finally, the quality of service offered by the NHS would be rigorously audited to ensure the best possible use of resources (linking back to the resource management initiative).

To achieve these goals, the NHS required an information revolution that extended the data collected by the resource management initiative so that costs could be more accurately measured, and prices set for services so they could form contracts in the new internal market for care. Capital assets were to be included in the pricing structures, and asset registers had to be collated for the first time in which, initially, every item of equipment in hospitals worth over £1,000 was logged and subjected to a financial accounting system through which depreciation could be recorded. This huge accounting exercise was justified on the grounds that hospitals had to be accountable for both their capital and non-capital costs in order to generate accurate, commercial prices for the contracting process.

To achieve the new status of self-governing trust, hospitals had to demonstrate that their senior professional staff were extensively involved in the management of their organisation, especially through its resource management. Consultants, regardless of their seniority, were to be made more accountable for their decision-making, and now had to strike:

> ... a proper balance between two legitimate pressures, both of which are focused on patients' interests: the professional responsibilities and rewards of the individual consultant; and the responsibility of managers to ensure that the money available for hospitals buys the best possible service for patients. (Secretary of State for Health, 1989, section 5.2)

Consultants were also required to work to fuller job descriptions than had been the case in the past, with distinction awards linked to their commitment to taking on managerial roles and for their role in the development of new services. Distinction award panels were no longer an entirely medical enclave, with the panels who decided them now including managers in an effort both to increase their accountability as well as to ensure that managerial involvement was rewarded.

GP practices with a patient list of over 11,000 were able to apply for 'fundholding' status, receiving a budget for referrals and diagnostic tests. The intention behind this was to move some of the contracting for care from district health authorities to doctors, who were regarded as the professionals closest to patients, their GPs, and to increase the power and status of referring GPs as a result. GP referral decisions, in fundholding surgeries, now carried resources with them, and this was seen as a means of incentivising hospitals to provide better service and to drive down waiting times. In turn, the government wanted to make it easier for patients to change GPs and to try and drive up standards in surgeries as well.

Importance of the internal market

The introduction of the internal market was important in that many of those proposals appeared on many fronts to represent a challenge to the underlying dynamics of the health service – giving managers greater authority through the market-based environment and increased access to formerly closed-off areas of medical control, such as pay awards. GP fundholders were meant to increase their power through resources being attached to their referral decisions, and patients become stronger through the ability to change their GPs more easily. But the introduction of the internal market was also important because of how it was formulated and conducted.

In the 1960s and 1970s it seemed unthinkable for the government to attempt healthcare reorganisation without extensive consultation with the medical profession. The first NHS reorganisation, in 1974, was the result of 10 years of debate including numerous government consultative documents, green and white papers. The mutually dependent, 'double bed' relationship with doctors meant that the government recognised that it depended heavily on the medical profession to implement its reorganisation. Equally, the status and popularity of the medical profession meant that its leaders were able to make direct appeals through the media and press to the public. Such actions could make life politically difficult for any government putting forward proposals with which the doctors did not agree. The British Medical Association and Royal Colleges were not just learned bodies, but, as the Thatcher government also suspected, deeply effective lobbying institutions that expected to have a significant role in any discussions about the future of the NHS.

The government effectively excluded medical representative groups from the discussions that put together the internal market proposals. Participants in the review were largely internal to government, with Kenneth Clarke only stepping outside of a small group of senior ministers (including the Prime Minister and Chancellor) to use a small group of potentially sympathetic doctors as a sounding board, and then, with them sworn to secrecy.

When the *Working for patients* proposals were published they received a furious reaction from doctors' representative groups. The British Medical Association led a high-profile and expensive campaign against the proposals, using posters showing bulldozers captioned 'Mr Clarke's proposals for the NHS', and leaflets in GP surgeries advising patients of problems with the reforms.

Kenneth Clarke, however, did not back down. Even though the Prime Minister appeared to get cold feet in the face of the expected opposition of the medical profession (Timmins, 1995a, 1995b), Clarke persisted, even apparently goading the doctors by suggesting that any discussions he had with them about reorganisation led to them 'reaching for their wallets', and was unwilling to pilot his proposals in test sites up and down the country before they were fully implemented because they would be subject to 'sabotage'.

At the beginning of the 1990s, then, health politics were in something of a toxic situation. Despite the government introducing a range of initiatives to change healthcare during the 1980s through general management, contracting out, resource management and quality initiatives, little seemed to have fundamentally changed, but it looked as if the NHS was about to enter a new era when market-based incentives would be introduced, and managers would have increased leverage for securing change, especially over doctors. At the very least, the government had shown that they were no longer going to consult with the medical profession about the content of healthcare reorganisation. Any further changes, however, depended on the internal market being implemented as planned.

The 'shared version' of health politics and organisation

Harrison, Hunter and Pollitt (and their co-authors) constructed a detailed synthesis of research carried out on the dynamics of the NHS at the end of the 1980s (see, for example, Harrison 1988; Harrison et al, 1990, 1992b; Pollitt et al, 1991a), making use initially of a device they call the 'shared version' of health politics. This provides us with a starting point for considering the NHS in 1990, as well as for assessing the effects of subsequent reorganisations.

The 'shared version' has nine dimensions in which health policy and politics has the following characteristics:

• incremental, so change is slow and narrow in scope;

- subject to partisan mutual adjustment, so that no individual actor or institution is able to dominate health politics;
- the medical profession tends to be predominant in the decision-making process in the NHS because of its ability to veto decisions or proposals that it does not like;
- lay health authority members are in a weak position compared to both clinicians and senior managers;
- 'consumer' organisations are in a weak bargaining position in relation to the NHS;
- central government provides little operational influence over the implementation of most of its policies, but does have the ability to change both the level and distribution of resources available for healthcare;
- health authority managers (and indeed health managers more generally) occupy largely reactive roles and so deal primarily with disputes rather than shaping the future direction of their organisations;
- the process of partisan mutual adjustment, especially in relation to change, is time-consuming and tends to result in inertia;
- the 'whole, complex and slow-moving edifice has been underpinned by an extremely durable political consensus' (Harrison et al, 1990, p 8).

The nine elements of the 'shared version' are summarised below, in Table 2.1.

Although the 'shared version' still serves as a good summary of health politics in the NHS during the 1980s, the proposed internal market reorganisation was a significant challenge to it. The reorganisation attempted to quickly (compared to previous policy negotiations) introduce a significant organisational change that, although it had continuities with general management and resource management (as Kenneth Clarke implied above), also introduced an entirely new dynamic – that of the marketplace of purchasers and providers. The review process that led to the internal market was not one of partisan mutual adjustment, in which careful and slow negotiation between the various interested parties was carried out, but instead came from a relatively closed review that made little or no attempt to consult with the doctors. The medical profession's traditional veto power over policy proposals it opposed was therefore certainly undermined – although, as we will see, whether such proposals could be implemented in the face of medical opposition remained more open to question.

Table 2.1: The 'shared version' of health politics

Incrementalism	Changes tend to be slow, and narrow in scope
Partisan mutual adjustment	No one actor or institution is able to dominate
Medical profession have veto power	Doctor representative bodies are able to prevent policy changes that might adversely affect doctors in the NHS
Lay health authority members in weak position compared to doctors or managers	Health services are run with little reference to external pressures or controls – 'introversion'
Health consumer groups are weak	Health consumer groups have become more concentrated, but still exert relatively little power over decision-making processes
The 'centre' has little operational control over implementation, but does have control over resource allocation and distribution	Central government has little control and little information about how health services are run, but does control the overall budget and how it is distributed regionally
Health authority managers are largely 'reactive'	Managerial roles tend to be about fire-fighting, diplomacy, conflict-avoidance and consensus-seeking
Complexity of system contributes to inertia	The vast size and complexity of health services combined with entrenched interest groups makes change very difficult
Durable political consensus	No government has challenged the 'double bed' relationship between the state and the medical profession (see above), and the NHS continues to be popular and supported by the public

As with the recommendations of the *NHS management inquiry*, the internal market proposals required managers to stop being reactive, and to become strategic in their approach in order to succeed in a competitive, market-based environment, which again, if it happened, would challenge the basis of medical power. The introduction of the market dynamic was also meant to strengthen the role of patients or health 'consumers', giving them a stronger role in decision-making.

The internal market arguably made little difference in terms of central government's lack of operational control over the NHS, but may well have attempted to make a virtue of this by introducing a market dynamic and requiring health managers to take more responsibility for driving forward improvements rather than depending on government.

Finally, the political consensus instigated by the NHS in the 1946 Act, especially the 'double bed' relationship between the state and doctors, appeared to be directly under challenge because of the lack of consultation over the proposals, and also because the market itself was meant to give managers additional legitimacy in challenging clinicians who were not changing their practices to suit the new market-based form of organisation. Health managers were not exactly becoming agents of the state in challenging medical power and leading the challenge of working in a competitive environment, but were certainly being asked to make services more efficient and responsive to patients' needs, and if that meant challenging doctors not willing to work in new ways, then that certainly formed part of the new agenda. The 'concordat' in which the state allocated funds to the NHS, and doctors decided how they would be best spent, appeared to have been discarded. (The extent to which the internal market succeeded in bringing about change to the degree the government appeared to think possible is explored in the next chapter.)

Conclusion

In 1990, the NHS was an organisation that had undergone a decade of change, but with apparently little real effect. It was also, however, on the cusp of potentially significant reorganisation. The period from 1948 to 1974 had been a time of remarkable continuity in NHS organisation despite the service receiving poor budgets in the 1950s, having to work in the turbulent economic times of the 1960s, and coping with a major structural reform that occurred in 1974 following an extensive period of debate. The Conservative government elected in 1979 removed a tier of organisation, and then instigated an NHS management inquiry and a range of initiatives which put managerial change at their core. The government appointed general managers, tried to get clinicians more engaged in management and make them more aware of the financial consequences of their decisions, contracting out ancillary and domestic services, and constrained prescribing to achieve better value for money. By the end of the decade, however, the Conservatives wanted to go further, and without consulting doctors in the way in which they had become accustomed, proposed the most radical reorganisation of the NHS in the service's history up to that point.

That the government took so long to embark on significant NHS reorganisation is partly a function of the service's popularity with the British public, partly due to the Labour opposition being able to claim to be the political 'party of the NHS', having created it in 1946 and never letting the Conservatives forget that they voted against the plans in Parliament in that year, and partly due to the sheer scale and difficulty of radically changing such a large and complex organisation, especially in terms of its potential to be a vote loser in an election. In other areas of the public sector (including social housing, gas and electricity) widespread privatisation had occurred, but the NHS remained, at the end of the 1980s, a publicly owned and provided, remarkably socialist, organisation. The changes that were to come were ideologically in keeping with those made to the electricity and gas industries, in trying to introduce competitive forces and through them, greater dynamism into healthcare, but on a far more limited scale.

So there was a range of important dynamics characterising the NHS in 1990 into which the internal market reorganisation was being introduced.

In terms of the political context, the government had significantly challenged the basis of its relationship with the medical profession that had been established in 1948. By introducing reorganisation without consultation, and in the face of considerable medical opposition when details of an internal market emerged, it seemed to have deliberately engineered a confrontation with the doctors. The internal market itself seemed to challenge medical autonomy by proposing a range of potentially far-reaching changes that gave managers greater authority over doctors in a market-driven environment, but also gave them involvement in areas formerly restricted to doctors only, such as pay awards. The reorganisation, by giving GP fundholders budgets, created the possibility of hospital consultants having to change their practices in order to attract GP referrals and contracts, challenging the historical hierarchy in medicine that placed hospital practice ahead of general practice by giving purchasing resources to the latter. The end result, with the medical profession's representative groups and the government apparently barely on speaking terms, was not one that appeared immediately conducive to achieving far-reaching organisational change.

If we consider the context from the perspective of ideas, we can see the dominant organisational principle through which the NHS had been run until the late 1980s, based on medical autonomy, also coming under considerable challenge from a more managerial approach that utilised the planned market for care as providing legitimacy for giving managers additional authority. At the same time, however, there were no real systems for measuring the performance of doctors or for assessing how well they were doing in their jobs, and so the scale of the managerial challenge they were facing was still rather unclear. What was apparent was that doctors were beginning to be expected to account for themselves to those outside of their own profession for the first time, even if there appeared to be few actual sanctions that could be applied should their performance be considered to be poor.

The context of health politics and organisation in 1990, then, was one that was politically contentious, and with the medical profession still having considerable control over NHS organisations, it was hard to see how a successful implementation of the proposed internal market was going to work. The next chapter reviews the research exploring what happened in the 1990s, before moving on to consider New Labour's approach to healthcare reorganisation between 1997 and 2010.

THREE

Reorganising the NHS, 1990–2010

Chapter Two explored the Conservative government's attempts to reorganise healthcare in the 1980s, taking this account up to the introduction of the internal market at the end of that decade.

Having outlined the political and ideational context into which the internal market was being introduced at the end of Chapter Two, we now consider the programme theory for it. How was the internal market meant to work?

This chapter first considers the programme theory of the effects of the 1990s internal market reorganisation, before taking the story on to the change in government in 1997and New Labour's various attempts to reorganise healthcare in the 2000s. Chapters Four and Five then consider the evidence from Labour's healthcare reorganisations, before turning to the coalition government's 2010 Health and Social Care Bill.

Purchaser–provider split and the internal market

The logic underlying the programme theory of the purchaser–provider split was that it would allow purchasers to use their funding decisions to reward good providers of care with contracts, giving all providers a funding incentive to improve the quality of their service, and creating the opportunity for successful services to expand (Day and Klein, 1991). The internal market was also meant to incentivise purchasers to find the best value and best quality care for the people they were serving. The government believed that the introduction of market-like governance into the NHS would improve its performance by increasing efficiency and productivity, while at the same time raising quality and reducing the wasted 'resources on excessive administration' (Le Grand, 1991, p 1262) that they regarded as coming from a traditional public sector bureaucracy. The internal market represented an internal or wholesale market (in contrast to New Labour's later external, retail market) in that NHS managers were supposed to be working on behalf of patients as their agents, rather than patients being responsible for driving the process of choosing care for themselves. Patients, however, had limited choice or say in their healthcare apart from through GP fundholding and a very limited number of 'extra contractual referrals' (ECRs), which were quasi-individual contracts rather than making use of the more usual block contacting process.

As such, the programme theory of the internal market was very much in line with economics-based theories in which principals act on behalf of their agents, with district health authorities and GP fundholders buying care on behalf of patients, providers competing to secure care contracts and the dynamic between purchasers and providers thought to be a mechanism for driving up efficiency and the quality of care as a result.

It is worth making clear that this programme theory was not based on research evidence – it was a reorganisation first based on a general assumption that extending competition into public services was the best way to reform them, and second on the appeal of the logic of economic competition, rather than being grounded in any particular empirical evidence.

Potential problems with the programme theory

In addition to the lack of research evidence underpinning the reorganisation and contextual problems outlined in Chapter Two – in particular the conflictual political context into which the reorganisation was introduced and the dominance of clinical (especially medical) autonomy at the local level of both hospitals and GP practices – the programme theory outlined above had additional problems that it needed to address in order to have any chance of working.

The introduction of the internal market required a radical improvement in the information systems available in the NHS so that costs (both revenue and capital) could be accurately measured, and outcome data could be published to enable purchasers to make 'well informed and unrestricted choices' (Bennett and Ferlie, 1996, p 49) in a marketplace which could responsively deal with patient needs by increasing the accountability of services through a market-based model in which successful providers were rewarded through additional contracts. Resource flows had to be redesigned to follow referral decisions, so that good providers could be rewarded for retaining and gaining contracts, requiring further transformation in the information system supporting the internal market. And the information system had to be put in place in a way that did not make the costs of contracting so substantial that they outweighed any benefits the new market system might achieve.

Even as the internal market was introduced, commentators suggested there were significant problems with its underlying programme theory. Hunter (1996) suggested that the aims of the reforms were based on 'faith' in market principles rather than knowledge of the dynamics of the NHS. Bennett and Ferlie (1996) argued that the reorganisation conflated the economist ideal of the perfect market, with 'quasi-markets' being created within the public sector, when the situation in the NHS, which was far closer to imperfect competition and where less than perfect information systems were found, was very different to the economists' ideal.

Even as the internal market was being implemented, the government, going through a change in Prime Minister and facing continued medical opposition, appeared to be backing down from its more radical features. Health commentators noticed the language of the reorganisation softening so that '"competition" turned into "contestability"' (Sheldon, 1990), and Kenneth Clarke was moved on from the health portfolio with more conciliatory figures brought in to implement the reforms. It seemed as if the government, two years from an election and with a new Prime Minister, was seeking a smooth transition to the new arrangements rather than a 'big bang' (Klein, 1995) package designed to transform the NHS, as it had originally envisaged.

By 1994, the government had published a framework for market management designed to stabilise the internal market (Ham, 1996) and to establish rules for the handling of mergers of both purchasers and providers. It emphasised the importance of coordination in the purchasing function, and made it clear that the internal market was now envisaged as a managed market rather than a dynamic, competitive marketplace for care.

What happened as a result of the internal market reorganisation?

One of the stated aims of the internal market was to increase NHS efficiency. It is hard, however, to claim that this was achieved through such means. In the 1980s, despite the lack of apparent success of the introduction of general managers and resource management initiative (see Chapter Two) in challenging clinical practice, the average length of stay for acute cases fell by 28 per cent, throughput of cases per bed increased by 47 per cent, and bed occupancy was kept at a near optimal 85 per cent (any higher than this and there is a risk of increased hospital acquired infection). At the same time as these achievements, the average cost per inpatient case fell by 10 per cent, and the UK spent half the gross national product (GNP) and a third of the dollars per capita that the US spent on healthcare (Light, 1992). Despite the performance of hospitals not being closely monitored during the 1980s, in 1989 compared to 1980, hospitals treated 16 per cent more inpatients, took care of 19 per cent more emergencies and carried out 73 per cent more outpatient surgery (Iliffe and Munro, 2000). While it is certainly the case that many of the gains were due to clinical innovations such as day surgery, they still represent an impressive series of efficiency improvements.

In contrast, the costs of setting up and running the internal market put the NHS at an immediate cost disadvantage compared to the previous decade. The cost of putting in place the necessary organisational changes amounted to at least £2 billion, and this was before any attempt at estimating the annual running costs was taken into account (Petchey, 1993). Therefore, any small increases in productivity achieved during the decade had to be offset against the higher transaction costs incurred (Klein, 1999). Implementation costs were well in excess of initial estimates, with £165 million being paid for managerial support, and the number of general and senior managers rising from 1,240 in 1988 to 20,010 in 1993, while the numbers of nurses and midwives fell by 12.4 per cent (Baggott, 1997) – although measuring staff changes in this way can be difficult because of regradings and job titles changing. Hospitals did seem to become more aware of the costs of treatment, even if attempts at performance management struggled with the limitations of systems that could only measure a limited range of activities (Likierman, 1993). However, if the internal market was meant to increase efficiency, it appeared to be a 'spectacular failure' (Iliffe and Munro, 2000, p 318).

The average cost of managing the internal market in a fundholding practice was between £60,000 and £80,000, or around 6 per cent of the total annual budget. Fundholders struggled to find a balance between having sufficient scale to exercise negotiating power over hospitals, while at the same time being small enough to be responsive and close to their patients (Le Grand et al, 1998). Instead of having flexible contracts that allowed purchasers to closely track quality and volume, block contracts were often used because there was so little data about cost and quality. Block contracting meant that there was a move to agree three- or five-year service agreements which left little scope for renegotiation and the use of alternative providers should poor performance occur, effectively creating local cartels in which there was relatively little threat of contracts being lost by incumbents.

Purchasers, rather than actively seeking alternative providers of care to drive up efficiency and quality, preferred to offer stability and continuity of care, and GPs were reluctant to refer to consultants whose work they did not know (Exworthy and Halford, 1998), meaning that even fundholding practices were often not the sites of innovation they were expected to be. Fundholding may have had an impact on the margins of care by allowing its practices to be more 'nimble' (Glennerster et al, 1994), and giving a means for patients they referred to jump waiting queues, but this can be seen as an inequity in which care was delivered more quickly.

The lack of dynamism in the majority of purchasing was further compounded by patients being reluctant to be referred to hospitals outside of their local areas. Given this, neither purchasers nor providers appeared to favour the competitive principles on which the market was premised. The information infrastructure on which a market mechanism depends was singularly lacking, and 'reduced the contracting process to a mere device for moving money around the system' (Bennett and Ferlie, 1996, p 64).

It appeared that, rather than money following patient and doctor choices, patients were following the contracts agreed by district health authorities (Enthoven, 2000), with purchasers put in a position where they could not financially destabilise hospitals because of the political problems this would cause, and hospitals unable to reduce costs because of the need to remain comprehensive providers of care across the full range of activities. In addition, teaching hospitals had to be sheltered from market discipline in order to maintain expensive medical training programmes with Royal Colleges that required minimum patient activity levels.

Ham's review of the internal market (1999) suggested that competition had little measurable impact, but with some change at the margins coming from some well-run fundholders which had managed to innovate and even offer minor surgery. These changes, however, were few and far between. The internal market appeared to have little effect on pay, with most labour contracts remaining centrally negotiated and so offering little scope for trusts to try and find new ways to incentivise their staff through new employment terms and conditions (Maynard, 1994).

In terms of patient involvement, there was little scope for patient or patient groups to be more involved in health decision-making as either members of the public or as choosers of care (Baggott, 1997). Performance information was not widely used for strategic decision-making, either by patients or commissioners (Vaughan and Higgs, 1995; Russell, 1998), with indicators being used as a periodic means of external control as league tables of hospital performance were published. These appeared to be targeted more at the public rather than as a means of exerting managerial control (Boland and Silbergh, 1996). But it was not entirely clear what individual citizens were meant to do with the information that the league tables presented – indeed, district health authorities appeared unsure what to do with the patient opinion surveys they conducted more generally (Harrison and Wistow, 1992). It seemed to be the case that the performance management system was generating more inefficiencies than gains (Propper, 1995, p 1686). The stated aim of the reorganisation in extending patient choice and driving improvements through stronger patient voice did not seem to have been achieved.

Finally, there is evidence of a decrease in the transparency of NHS management and a reduction in accountability. The complexity of contracting arrangements made financial conduct more difficult to scrutinise, but audit processes led to the discovery of examples of fraud and waste, such as those found in the Wessex Computer Integration Scheme and which were due to unauthorised payments being made by senior managers (Baggott, 1997).

Summarising the effects of the internal market

The internal market reorganisation was costly to introduce, and appears to have led to a significant increase in the cost of managing the NHS, even if we allow for some clinical staff being regraded into managerial roles but continuing to practice as healthcare professionals. GP fundholding may have had benefits for some patients where innovative practices used the reorganisation to their advantage, but this also led to concerns that a 'two-tier' system of GP practices was being set up which went against the universalist principles of the NHS. Such benefits may not have exceeded the infrastructural and transaction cost of putting in place the market for care in the first place. There simply did not appear to be much of a marketplace for care (West, 1998), with a lack of competition, and a great deal of contracting being based on block agreements that reduced the potential for care contracts being moved to alternative providers in the face of poor performance.

Impact of the internal market on doctors in hospitals

Despite all the organisational change involved in introducing the internal market, the predominant organisational culture in the NHS remained clinical (Boyett and Finlay, 1995). Even where managers attempted to challenge clinicians, they often found themselves attempting to bridge the different medical 'tribes' (Hunter, 1996), with doctors remaining largely uninterested in the resource and cost issues involved in their practice (Kitchener, 1997).

The conflict between the medical profession and the government at the beginning of the reorganisation appeared to have resulted in clinicians disengaging from the reorganisation process, retaining control over its implementation even if medical representative groups had lost control of the policy-making process. Doctors continued to dominate the organisational arenas they regarded as most important (Laughlin, 1991). In 1995 the Audit Commission noted the lack of progress in tightening doctors' job descriptions to make them more accountable for their work, and consultants were criticised for continuing to engage in private work when they attended only 54 per cent of their fixed NHS sessions (Audit Commission, 1995). Managers seemed to be struggling to find ways to make doctors more accountable (McGucken, 1994; Richards, 1998). Most doctors continued to believe that medical malpractice should be resolved with the profession only (Brearley, 1996), even in the face of criticisms about doctors' inability to self-regulate adequately (Donaldson, 1994; Sandford, 2001).

Doctors tended to regard audit as a means by which the government attempted to control and discipline them, and in the hierarchical professional medical setting, peers were reluctant to criticise one another (Black and Thompson, 1993). Even after medical audit became mandatory for doctors, it remained professionally rather than managerially run (Pollitt, 1993; Packwood et al, 1994).

Doctors appeared both reluctant to have their work overseen by non-medically qualified managers, but at the same time reluctant to enter managerial roles themselves. Those doctors who worked in clinical directorates regarded them more as a means of blocking the decisions of non-clinical managers than as a means of improving services through collaboration (Salter, 1999). Only a minority of clinical directors were committed to their managerial role because they could not see how the post would lead to a senior management position, and because they regarded their roles as ones in which they were only 'part-time' managers (Riordan and Simpson, 1994). Clinical directorates appeared too often to generate parallel managerial structures rather than being integrated into NHS line management, with clinical directors remaining wary of activities that might distance them from their clinical colleagues (Marnoch et al, 2000).

Impact of the internal market on nursing

Despite the continued problems with nurse education and recruitment in the 1990s, new nursing roles did offer the opportunity for existing staff to expand their expertise and enhance their professional status in primary care (Lempp, 1995; Broadbent, 1998), and in hospitals nurses often led quality-based initiatives, seeing them as an opportunity to improve patient care. Many of the new directors of quality assurance came from nursing backgrounds (Pollitt, 1993), resulting in this area being one in which nursing could provide a lead.

Impact of the internal market on GPs

As noted above, fundholding did lead to some innovation, with proactive GPs able to change referral patterns and drive improvements in local health areas, albeit giving rise to concerns about 'two-tier' services emerging where non-fundholding GPs were unable to achieve the same outcomes. More generally, however, fundholding led to problems of coordination as district health authorities (the major single purchasers of care) had no means of coordinating fundholders in their local areas, and so found it difficult to plan care purchasing around them. It seemed that the move to more fragmented, market-based governance led to particular problems in areas such as London, which required government intervention to prevent the purchaser–provider split leading to hospital closure, and in treatment areas such as cancer, which required a national plan to make sure the best care was widely available (Baggott, 1997). It seemed as if the government was prepared to revert to central planning where either the outcome of the purchaser–provider split looked as if it might prove politically unacceptable (as in London, where it might have led to hospital closure), or where it could not meet the aims of government policy (as in the case of cancer services, which required a higher level of coordination). The purchaser–provider split, therefore, was never regarded as a market for care in the manner in which economists would understand it, but was instead highly managed and controlled according to government political priorities.

The 'shared version' after the internal market reorganisation

The 'shared version' gives us a means of exploring the effects of the internal market on the starting position in 1990s, and of establishing the context of care at the end of the Conservative's time in office in 1997.

The Conservatives had taken a confrontational approach to policy-making during the formulation and introduction of the internal market, but this seemed to lead to substantial implementation problems because of the need to get the, by then angry and disengaged, medical profession to cooperate to make the reorganisation a success. The reorganisation was introduced into a politically confrontational context that did not make for an easy implementation of a complex and challenging programme of changes. The government can be seen to have retreated from its original plan, with changes in Prime Minister and Secretary of State for Health leading to a more conciliatory approach, giving those who were responsible for implementing the reorganisation on the ground less authority than they might otherwise have had, and with the reorganisation initially emphasising 'smooth take off' rather than the significant challenge to the medical profession it might have been.

In addition to the difficulties of getting the medical profession to implement a reorganisation whose introduction they had campaigned against, in a context where governments had generally struggled to secure any kind of significant change as a result of reorganising the NHS, there were several other factors that limited the potential for change in the 1990s. The real lack of competition in the internal market was due to the limited number of alternative providers of care in many areas, and a general reluctance from the public to travel far when referred on from their GP surgeries. Equally, purchasers of care seemed reluctant to refer patients to different providers, especially those they did not have established relationships with, and the use of block contracts severely limited the potential for any kind of market to develop (Exworthy and Peckham, 2006).

The end result was a 'becalming' (Wainwright, 1998) of health politics during the mid to late 1990s in which collaboration replaced competition as the main means by which the NHS was meant to improve. There was some evidence of proactive GPs finding ways of changing the dynamics of their local health areas where fundholders were able to find new patterns of referrals, but achieving large-scale, systemic change proved elusive (Greener and Mannion, 2009b).

It seems reasonable to conclude, then, at the end of the 1990s, that the 'shared version' remained remarkably intact despite ten years of concerted attempts at change from the Conservative governments. Although policy-making had shown a break from the 'slow-moving consensus' of the past, in which the doctors expected to be extensively consulted, the implementation of the internal market had proved to be rather less radical than expected. Hospital consultants retained a significant degree of autonomy, able to opt out of, or minimally comply with, initiatives based around quality improvement, and unwilling to take on management roles that they felt might compromise their ability to practice medicine. Health managers struggled to use the purchaser–provider split as a means of challenging medics in an environment where consultants often showed little interest in, or even open disdain towards, them, and the government appeared to lose interest in its own reorganisation agenda after 1990 under a new Prime Minister with more pressing political issues to face in his own party. In the 1990s, Secretaries of State such as William Waldegrave and Virginia Bottomley appeared less driven to attempt to radically reorganise healthcare, and more concerned with getting existing structures to work.

GPs, where they were proactive fundholders, achieved some modest gains where they were able to offer new services, offer their patients reduced waiting times or move care contracts to alternative providers, but these changes were limited in scope by the small size of practice budgets and the lack of incentives for consultants to protect old contracts or pursue new ones because of their own secure employment tenure. Nurses in both hospitals and GP surgeries took on new roles, often with notable success, but did not appear to see a significant increase in their professional standing, and with extended responsibilities often perceived as being the 'gift' of doctors giving up responsibilities they no longer wished to hold (Broadbent, 1998).

In 1996, a year before they were to lose a general election to 'New Labour', the Conservative government issued a remarkably conciliatory White Paper celebrating the success of the NHS rather than promising more organisational change (Secretary of State for Health, 1996). The road from 1989 and *Working for patients* had seen the government move away from proposing a radical, market-driven model to one in which partnership working was celebrated. The political consensus central to the NHS appeared to have undergone a serious challenge at the beginning of the decade by the government overtly taking on the doctors at the national policy level, even if the subsequent reforms made little difference for most medics in their everyday work. However, the government had successfully challenged the political concordat between the medical profession and the state after *Working for patients*. Even if it subsequently did not implement its proposals in a radical way, the government had shown it could change the organisation of the NHS in the face of opposition from the doctors (Greener, 2002). However, in that process it had expended a great deal of political capital and energy, and seemed to lack the will to implement the reorganisation in anything like its original form.

The political context, then, appeared to be rather calmer in 1997 than in 1990, but with each side left chastened by the impact of health policy in the 1990s. The government had learned that it may well be able to make policy and introduce legislation in the face of medical opposition, but also that it would struggle to implement radical new policy in the face of medical opposition. The medical profession had learned that they could no longer expect to be automatically consulted in NHS policy-making, with their public campaign against the internal market failing to prevent it being introduced. However, the less-than-radical implementation of the internal market and the continued ability of doctors to operate with high degrees of autonomy in hospitals and GP surgeries meant that little change appeared to have taken place where healthcare was actually delivered.

In terms of the ideational context, the changes of the 1990s had forced doctors and other clinicians to begin to adopt a new language around budgets and efficiency savings, even if that language had not yet intruded into their everyday practices as far as the government might have wished. Even though doctors were resisting the intrusion of managerial discourse into their practice, and were often very effective in preserving their clinical autonomy, they were also having to accept that the way they had to describe their work was gradually changing. The number of managers in the NHS was increasing, and clearer lines of accountability, no matter how poorly enforced, were put in place. Ideationally, the internal market did not change the NHS into a managerial institution, but did begin to create the means for a more significant challenge to clinical autonomy in the 2000s and 2010s as managerial language, and managerial practices and technologies, gradually became more accepted as part of everyday life.

Health policy under New Labour, 1997–2010

During the general election of 1997, Labour campaigned on the basis of 'saving the NHS', also making a pledge to reduce waiting lists, and to abolish the Conservative's internal market. On their election, the intention was to heal the 'wounds' with the medical profession 'reduce inequalities, and install a cooperative model of commissioning for health gain' (Light, 1998, p 217).

Labour inherited an NHS with the internal market still in place, but as noted above, it was largely moribund and had gradually been overlaid by guidance requiring a collaborative approach to contracting, where three- to five-year block contracts were the norm. After a radical period of health policy, incrementalism had re-established itself, the doctors largely retained their clinical autonomy, health consumer groups remained weak, and although managers had by now a range of additional tools and mechanisms for measuring care performance, these were not being systemically used to drive improvements and change. There seemed to be little political appetite from either Labour or the Conservatives for further radical healthcare reorganisation.

On returning to power, Labour quickly published a White Paper to reveal its plans for healthcare (Secretary of State for Health, 1997). The tone was conciliatory. Labour claimed to have abolished the internal market on the grounds that it represented a bureaucratic waste, with primary care groups (PCGs) being set up to take over from the internal market commissioning (purchasing) organisations, and fundholding abolished amid concerns over its 'two-tier' outcomes (see above). Contracts were moved to longer-term service agreements to attempt to reduce the transaction costs of the NHS, and to save £250 million per year. Despite Labour's claims, the internal market was not abolished, but rather moved onto an even more cooperative and longer-term basis (Powell, 1998; Iliffe and Munro, 2000). Labour attempted to achieve greater cross-service and cross-boundary working by requiring the establishment of local Health Improvement Programmes, and establishing Health Action Zones in particularly deprived areas (Matka et al, 2002).

There were also signs, however, of the government wanting to control the NHS more firmly from the centre. Labour proposed a system in which there would be national standards of care to try and achieve greater equality of service access (Butler and Roland, 1998), raising some concerns about a possible tendency towards greater centralisation (Klein and Maynard, 1998). These concerns were added to by the creation of the National Institute for Clinical Excellence (NICE)[1] to regulate the introduction of new drugs and treatments into the NHS on the basis of whether they were cost-effective as well as clinically effective (Peckham et al, 2005).

Between 1997 and early 2000, Labour's initial period of policy-making formed a distinct phase that developed the proposals in the 1997 White Paper, and is summarised in Table 3.1 below.

Table 3.1: Timeline for Labour policy, 1997 to early 2000

Year	Events	Legislation and documentation
1997	March: NHS (Primary Care) Bill receives Royal Assent May: general election, in which Labour gains majority and forms a new government under Tony Blair	*The new NHS: Modern, dependable* NHS (Primary Care) Act NHS (Private Finance) Act *Designed to care: Renewing the National Health Service in Scotland*
1998	Abolition of GP fundholding	Scotland Act Government of Wales Act *Information for health: An information strategy for the modern NHS, 1998- 2005* *A first class service: Quality in the new NHS* *Modernising social services*
1999	PCGs (481) Clinical Standards Board for Scotland National Institute for Clinical Excellence (NICE) Commission for Health Improvement (CHI) Walk-in NHS centres National framework for mental health services Devolution of power to Scotland and Wales	Health Act *Saving lives: Our healthier nation*
2000	Abolition of the NHS Executive Primary care trusts (PCTs) (first wave) – national service frameworks Food Standards Agency	*The NHS Plan*

Source: Compiled from Ham (2000) and NHS Reform (www.sochealth.co.uk/news/NHSreform.htm)

By 2000, however, a new direction for health policy and organisation seemed to be appearing. First, Health Secretary, Frank Dobson (an 'old Labour' figure in many respects), had made what proved to be an unsuccessful attempt to become Mayor of London and was replaced by Alan Milburn. Second, Labour found itself criticised for the lack of progress it was making in improving healthcare, even from its own supporters (Giddens, 2002). Third, the pledge it had made to reduce waiting times in 1997 appeared to be at risk, requiring the government to address the NHS as a potential problem area (Baggott, 2006).

In 2000, Milburn put together the NHS Plan, which ambitiously provided a framework for the next 10 years to modernise care. Milburn appears to have largely constructed the document himself, but was wise enough to make sure a range of senior NHS figures both saw and endorsed it before publication. This meant that the government could present the NHS Plan as the result of extensive consultation rather than the imposition of government ideology, as the medical profession had described *Working for patients* in 1989 (Klein, 2006). The NHS Plan presented the NHS as being a '1940s system operating in a 21st century world' (Secretary of State for Health, 2000, p 2), and claimed this led to a number of problems including underfunding, a lack of national standards, barriers between services, disempowered patients and over-centralisation.

To confront these problems, the NHS Plan proposed:

- the introduction of a system of inspection and accountability for all parts of the NHS. These standards aimed to combine national standards with greater local autonomy, with new funding available and potentially greater exemption from inspection to reward high-performing organisations;
- a new consultant contract that aimed to give most money to the doctors working hardest in the NHS;
- that nurses and other health professionals would be given bigger roles in line with their qualifications and expertise;
- that local health services and local social services would be brought closer together in one organisation;
- that the NHS and the private sector would work more closely together, not just to build new hospitals (through the private finance initiative [PFI]) but also to provide NHS patients with the operations they needed;
- that patients would have an advocate in every hospital, so that a system designed around patients was one with more power for patients.

The NHS Plan began a period of hyperactive healthcare reorganisation (Smith et al, 2001) that was to have profound consequences for those working in the health service.

Performance management

As noted in Chapter Two, performance indicators in the 1980s and 1990s were used primarily as a means of constructing league tables, but appeared to have the public as their main audience, with low performers facing castigation from the local media (Vaughan and Higgs, 1995; Russell, 1998). Performance measures were not really used as an internal managerial tool. By the 2000s, the government's tendencies to want to exert central control to help targets over waiting lists be reached, and so to show real progress in delivering change in the NHS, were reinforced by high-profile medical scandals which appeared to suggest existing devolved audit processes were not working adequately. National standards were to be developed for all major conditions that were a mix of clinical targets and patient-led indicators, such as, by 2004, being able to see a primary care professional within 24 hours and a GP within 48 hours.

The new approach to performance management for hospitals was the most visible example of central government taking a far stronger role in the day-to-day workings of the NHS. From a situation in the 1960s where health ministers complained of having virtually no information about the workings of the health service to be able to exert any kind of control (Powell, 1966), the technological revolution created the possibility for huge data sets to be gathered about the workings of hospitals, and for them to be compared to standards set by the government, as well as for performance comparisons to be made between hospitals.

The introduction of clinical governance in 2001 meant that board members of health organisations were now responsible for both the clinical and managerial aspects of care (CHI, 2001). Clinical governance was an important idea in the early 2000s, with Chief Medical Officer, Liam Donaldson, its chief architect, and was a further attempt to get clinicians and managers to work together more closely by integrating responsibilities and accountabilities. NHS trusts were to choose clinicians to lead clinical governance and to set up action plans to deliver high-quality care, but the guidance was not prescriptive as to exactly how this was meant to happen. The intention was to create 'a systematic set of mechanisms that will support staff and develop all health organisations to deliver a new approach to quality' (DH, 1999).

In primary care, the introduction of the Quality and Outcomes Framework (QOF) for GP practices led to them having to demonstrate they were achieving 'points' against pre-defined quality standards to both drive up standards and recognise practices' achievements (Gunstone, 2007). The QOF was designed to change the basis of remuneration for GPs to incentivise them to provide high-quality, evidence-based care, and was a central part of the new General Medical Services (GMS) contract introduced in 2004. Achievement was measured against a range of evidence-based indicators, with points and payments awarded according to level of achievement. There was also to be a bigger role for GPs in shaping local services. More would become GPs with special interests (GPSIs), able to perform minor surgery within general practice (as some enterprising GP fundholders had done in the 1990s).

The introduction of performance management in hospitals and the QOF in GP practices makes up the central plank of the emergence of a new programme theory for healthcare improvement in which centrally set standards were put in place, and the performance of local health organisations in meeting them monitored. The idea was to put in place rewards for good performance, and sanctions for those falling short of the standards required. In the case of the performance management system, additional freedoms from inspection were to be given to hospitals measured as achieving high performance (through 'earned autonomy'), but alongside this was also the threat of increased inspection and even managerial teams being replaced wholesale if they were measured as being poor performers. In the case of the QOF, high performers stood to achieve higher levels of funding (as well as the status of exceeding their 'points' targets), and poor performers cuts in their budgets.

Institutional changes

In 2003 the Health and Social Care (Community Health and Standards) Act was published that established a new kind of healthcare organisation – foundation trusts. These were providers of care within the NHS, but (similarly to the role played by NHS trusts in *Working for patients*) were to be given a greater range of freedoms and power to manage their own affairs compared to standard NHS trusts through systems of earned autonomy. They would be able to access new sources of capital, invest surpluses in the development of new services, tailor their governance arrangements to the needs of local communities, and be overseen by a new independent regulator called Monitor, which could intervene where significant problems arose. It was also intended that they would have closer links with their communities and so develop services tailored accordingly (DH, 2005).

The extension of nursing roles that had gathered pace in the 1990s was to continue. The NHS Plan invited more nurses to become leaders, as 'There are simply too few of them' (Secretary of State for Health, 2000, p 90). By 2004 there were to be around 1,000 nurse consultants. These would 'work with senior hospital doctors, nurses and midwives in drawing up local clinical and referral protocols alongside primary care colleagues' (p 86). Modern matrons were to be introduced to work in hospital wards with special responsibilities for the politically sensitive area of infection control, tackling public concerns about the spread of viruses such as MRSA (Methicillin-resistant Staphylococcus aureus).

The Commission for Health Improvement (CHI) was set up to make regular inspections of health bodies with the aim of improving the quality of care in NHS hospitals, community and primary care services. Annual publication of the results of the Performance Assessment Framework was now CHI's responsibility. It also could make inspections for hospital cleanliness.[2] Every NHS organisation was to be inspected by the CHI every four years, and any organisations rated 'red' under the traffic light system (which in implementation became a 'star'-based system, before that too was changed) could be reinspected every two years. The CHI could also be sent into organisations where there was concern over poor healthcare or patient safety. The CHI and Audit Commission were also expected to carry out national inspections and reports. Following the Report of the Public Inquiry into children's heart surgery at the Bristol Royal Infirmary, 1984–95, the inspection role for the CHI was strengthened to try and give the public independent assurance that each provider of NHS services had proper quality assurance, and that it had adequate quality improvement mechanisms in place. A statutory duty was placed on chief executives and service managers to be accountable for quality, and the National Patient Safety Agency (NPSA) was created to establish a single national system of reporting and analysis of adverse medical events and near-misses.

From 2000, then, health policy appeared to be moving to a model where greater government control was being exerted over the NHS, challenging the element of the shared version that suggests that policy-makers actually had very little control over implementation (or 'delivery'). Care frameworks and the establishment of bodies such as the CHI put in place new structures and organisations that were primarily about trying to increase central control. The introduction of the Performance Assessment Framework in hospitals, and the QOF in GP surgeries, demanded computer-based information systems could (at least theoretically) measure the activities of clinicians and managers. The government wanted to make use of these systems in their plans to modernise healthcare by delivering on political promises to reduce waiting lists. The 'central control' programme theory, as we will refer to it, was a means of attempting to get local healthcare organisations to work to central targets through the use of a top-down control system in which high performers were to be rewarded, and poor performers subject to sanctions.

Patient choice and the creation of a mixed economy of care

In addition to the introduction of a programme of reorganisation that attempted to exert greater central control over the day-to-day workings of the NHS, after 2000 Labour also began, through a gradual and piecemeal approach, to re-establish a marketplace for healthcare. In 2001, the government published a consultative document titled *Extending choice for patients* (DH, 2001b), which provided the first sign that market-based mechanisms were once again finding favour with government. In London, a pilot project was run in which long-waiting patients were given the option of either choosing a new provider of care or continuing to wait, with the majority choosing to move their care somewhere else (Coulter et al, 2005). This preference to move to a new provider of care rather than face longer waiting times was seen as a sign by the government that offering patients more choice was potentially popular with patients, as well as a means of achieving a basis for patients leading organisational change if resources could be made to follow their choices. A new computer system, 'Choose and Book', was put in place to try and provide the information system infrastructure to move care appointments out of the control of consultants and either into GP surgeries or through the use of call centres as a means of moving referral appointments more in line with patient wishes.

To strengthen the motivation of providers to attract patients, the government wanted a system where funds followed patient choices. But wary of providers engaging in cost-based competition to try and attract care referrals, the government effectively fixed prices by setting a 'national tariff' which varied by condition and severity of condition. This meant that the new market for care, in common with the 1990s internal market, was attempting to put in place a logic in which the best providers of care would be rewarded through increased resources following patient and GP choices. The new system for rewarding referrals was known as 'Payment by Results' (PbR) (DH, 2002).

In contrast to the internal market of the 1990s, the government made it a central part of their approach to the new 'mixed economy of care' to extend the use of not-for-profit and private providers to increase both the capacity of the system as a whole and to increase competition, to drive up responsiveness, raise efficiency and improve quality (Warner, 2011).

As such, the new market for care was not 'internal', or 'quasi' as it had been in the 1990s, as it was not just about public providers competing with one another. Instead, it aimed to get new entrants from the private and not-for-profit sectors to compete for care with existing public providers.

The new 'mixed economy of care' therefore attempted to address two of the central criticisms made of the 1990s model: that there was not enough competition to make the market work, and that providers could undercut one another on price, which was a threat to care quality. These criticisms were to be dealt with by extending competition to non-public providers, and by fixing the price of care.

By 2006, the mixed economy of care had reached a point where patients were to be offered a choice of provider whenever they were being referred on for care by their GP, and indeed to choose the GP who could best provide primary care for them in the first place (DH, 2006; Green, 2006). To address concerns about the availability of good information in the 1990s, the government invested in the 'NHS Choices' website to try and give patients support in making the new choices being offered to them, and leaflets were produced with basic comparative data about the main providers of care in each area.

Alongside changes based on choice and competition, the government also sought to encourage patients to enter the NHS through new routes, putting in place NHS Direct (a web and telephone-based system to provide advice to the public), through NHS 'walk-in' centres, which would provide primary care services that were more convenient for patients to access than seeing their own GPs, as well as often experimenting with nurse-led organisations, The intention was to give patients a choice not only when they required care from the NHS (through a choice of a provider in the referral process), but also in how they accessed the NHS in the first place.

As such, alongside the 'central control' set of initiatives designed to get health services to 'deliver' (Barber, 2007) on targets set by the government, a second series of changes to health service organisation seemed to reveal a gradually phasing and layering (Mays et al, 2011) of initiatives designed to put in place a marketplace for care that was more robust and dynamic than the 'internal' market of the 1990s.

The programme theory for the new mixed economy of care was a modified version of what it had been in the earlier decade. Providers were to compete for contracts (as some centralising of that process had to take place), and also for individual GP and patient choices within those contracts as the PbR system was more fine-grained than the block contracting approach of the 1990s. Instead of there simply being public providers attempting to compete for contracts, there was now to be a greater range of public and non-public providers competing in the marketplace for care, increasing competition, and so making gains in responsiveness and efficiency more possible, and raising the standard of care as a result. To get purchasers and providers to focus on quality rather than price (the 1990s internal market had allowed contract negotiation over both), prices were centrally set.

The new mixed economy of health forms a key part of the 'local dynamic' programme theory in place in the 2000s. The 'local' element of 'local dynamic' endeavours to capture the attempt to achieve improvement through the interaction of individual organisations in the new marketplace for care, rather than through the imposition of central standards and targets. 'Dynamic' is used as the reorganisations were meant to drive improvement by generating the need for services to be adapted in line with competitive forces or service user need rather than subject to continual central government interference. Although the marketplace for care was imposed through central policy-making, it was meant to work at the local level without continual government involvement − hence it represented a different, but parallel, series of reorganisations compared to the 'central control' changes, even if both often appeared to be introduced at the same time with little coordination between the two.

Patient and public involvement in the NHS

The second part of the programme theory of 'local dynamic' reorganisation was concerned with achieving greater patient and public involvement (PPI) outside of the expansion of patient choice in the new market for healthcare. In the 1990s, as we saw above, little progress seemed to have been made in achieving greater patient involvement in health services, either in citizen-type roles, where they could get involved in local health organisations, or in consumer-type roles, where they could make choices and expect complaints to be acted on (Baggott, 1997).

In 1999, the government announced its intention of making PPI a central value of the NHS, both at the collective level by involving the public more in planning and strategy, but also requiring patients to be more extensively consulted in individual decisions about their care. The NHS Plan (Secretary of State for Health, 2000) put in place a range of agencies to these ends, and the Health and Social Care Act 2001 made it a duty of NHS bodies to consult the public in both the planning and operation of health services (Hughes et al, 2009). The community health councils established in the 1970s were abolished (among some controversy from their advocates) and replaced by patient and public involvement forums (PPIFs) managed by the Commission for Patient and Public Involvement in Health (CPPIH). The PPIFs were also expected to coordinate their activity with local government overview and scrutiny committees in an attempt to combine elected democratic representation with healthcare monitoring.

The creation of foundation trusts and councils of governors offered an opportunity for the public to become 'members' of the new organisations, and was seen by some commentators as providing a means by which the NHS might become a more mutually run institution with greater democratic involvement (Birchall, 2003). But others saw it as a rather weak attempt to achieve greater public involvement from which little real change would result (Klein, 2003).

In 2003, the Health and Social Care (Community Health and Standards) Act gave the Healthcare Commission (formally the Commission for Healthcare Audit and Inspection) the responsibility of conducting patient surveys and making sure patient groups were consulted in local service planning and provision, and the Patient Advice and Liaison Service (PALS) took over the roles formerly overseen by community health councils in supporting complainants and giving patients the right to redress over cancelled operations. A national Patient Survey was put in place, and financial rewards offered for organisations that performed well on it. Lay membership was increased on the General Medical Council, the NHS Modernisation Board and on NICE (the treatment-overseeing body). Then, in 2007, the government abolished PPIFs and replaced them with local involvement networks (LINks), although with the new body apparently having a very similar role.

The continual reorganisation of PPI mechanisms in the NHS does appear to show that the government was serious in trying to achieve a stronger voice for groups other than clinicians and managers in the running of health services. It represents a second strand of the 'local dynamic' programme theory that attempts to work by getting healthcare organisations to put patient concerns more centrally in their day-to-day workings through 'voice' mechanisms which were designed to work alongside the 'choice'-based mechanisms put in place in the mixed economy of care.

PPI was meant to work by healthcare organisations listening to patients more closely, addressing public concerns about healthcare services, and responding to complaints more effectively. As with the reinstatement of the market for care, although these changes were centrally imposed by the government, they were designed to put in place a 'local dynamic' in which improvements to health services would be made on a self-sustaining basis through the interactions between health organisations, patients and the public, rather than through the setting of central standards and monitoring against them (the central control programme theory above).

When combined with the reinstatement of the market for care, the full local dynamic programme theory emerges in which local healthcare organisations (both public and non-public) compete with one another to secure contracts through GP and patient choices, and with all healthcare organisations taking local patient and public wishes seriously by incorporating them into the design and running of their services, dealing with complaints effectively and problems seriously, and so improving their efficiency, responsiveness and care standard. All this was to be achieved without the need for central government to continually interfere in their running.

In all, then, the period up to 2010 saw the introduction of a new mixed economy of care in which public and non-public providers were to be cast in increasingly competitive-type relationships. There was a range of attempts at getting both patients and the public more involved in running their local health services. The combination of 'choice' and 'voice' was meant to put in place a new dynamic designed to make health services 'self-improving'.

Conclusion

By the time the Conservative government left office in 1997 it seemed as if they were no longer interested in radical reform in healthcare. The change in Prime Minister in 1990, and the subsequent changes in the Secretary of State for Health, meant that the internal market never was much of a market, and the government appeared to become more concerned with other areas of policy-making, especially in the post-1992 period in which it faced a much-reduced majority and a range of internal political difficulties. By 1996 the government seemed to be advocating an approach to the NHS that was as much based on partnership and collaboration as on market-based mechanisms.

On returning to power in 1997, Labour appeared, on the one hand, to go through a period in which they largely continued with the direction of Conservative health policy in the middle 1990s, moving further away from the market by making contracts more long term and by abolishing fundholding, but on the other hand, putting in place new institutions that held the potential to exert a great deal more central control over healthcare. By 2000, frustration seemed to be building that improvement in the NHS was proving elusive, and that waiting list promises in the 1997 election manifesto might be missed. The result was the NHS Plan, which increased the command and control thinking evident in earlier policy changes through, among other centralising changes, the introduction of a performance management regime. After this, the subsequent reintroduction of the market (complete with new providers from the non-public sector and fixed prices) meant that the 2000s were a period of almost continual reorganisation.

The government appeared to be attempting to drive change from the centre by introducing agencies to exert control over the monitoring of health services, as well as through deciding what treatments the NHS could provide, but also gradually reintroducing programmes of change based on trying to get local organisations to respond in a more dynamic way through the use of market-based mechanisms and by repeated attempts to achieve greater PPI in the NHS. It is hard to see how all these changes form a consistent (or sometimes even coherent) approach to reorganising healthcare, and it sometimes appeared as if the government had become a consumer of policy, and impatient for change, switching from one idea to the next without properly implementing any of them or allowing time to see what worked and what did not (Hunter, 2008).

Despite the difficulties of assessing health reform in such a hyperactive period of policy-making, we can try to assess the success (or otherwise) of Labour's efforts in terms of their attempts to drive change from the centre, especially through its Performance Assessment Framework and the QOF in GP surgeries. Local dynamic changes, in contrast, were driven through the need to compete in the new marketplace for care, and to take more seriously the demand to treat patient and public needs more seriously (Greener, 2009; Greener and Powell, 2009).

The next chapter explores the dynamics of central control, and local dynamic programme theories in more depth, as well as exploring what research says about how well these attempts at reorganisation worked, and what we can learn from them for the NHS of the 2010s.

Notes

[1] NICE has since undergone a number of name changes, with the nearest present body being the National Institute for Health and Care Excellence.

[2] The CHI has since undergone a number of name changes, with the nearest present body being the Care Quality Commission (CQC).

FOUR

'Central control' reorganisation in the NHS in the 2000s

The context of health policy in the 2000s

Attempting to reorganise the NHS so that there is a stronger means of managing the performance of healthcare organisations is not a new idea. Performance indicators were first introduced in the 1970s and were extended during the 1980s, with the first comprehensive national performance data set disseminated in September 1983 to local health authorities in a series of 'grey books' (Pollitt, 1985). In 1991, and marking the creation of the internal market, these performance indicators were relabelled health service indicators. By the end of the decade their use was still largely an 'external' exercise where ratings were published once a year and league tables constructed, apparently mostly with the public (or at least the media) as their intended audience, but with few penalties for NHS trusts rated as the worst performers, and few rewards for those graded as performing well.

This chapter considers how Labour put in place a series of organisational changes based around the goal of achieving greater 'central control' over implementation (or 'delivery', as it became known) during the 2000s. It considers the use of performance management systems in both hospitals and GP surgeries, but with, we will argue, very important differences that affected the relative successes of such systems in those different contexts. Because the context here has already been outlined to some extent in Chapter Three, there is necessarily some repetition in order both to be clear about the policy environment of the 2000s, but also to try and make each chapter as free-standing as possible in terms of content. We hope that presenting the material in this way adds to clarity without putting readers off.

As noted in Chapter Three, there were signs from 1997 and 1998 that Labour wanted to tighten central control over policy implementation, but it was not until the publication of the NHS Plan in 2000 (Secretary of State for Health, 2000) that the new direction became fixed. The NHS Plan marked the beginning of a period of increased investment in the NHS, raising the proportion of gross domestic product (GDP) spent on healthcare in the UK to around the European Union (EU) average from being around 2 percentage points below. The Wanless Report into health financing (Wanless, 2002) further emphasised the need for an increase in healthcare expenditure, and was crucial in setting an historically unprecedented increase in funding for the NHS. Despite the hyperactive nature of Labour's reorganisations during the decade, they are almost certain to be regarded as a 'golden age' in terms of the availability of resources (Bevan, 2011). The increase in funding, however, meant that the mantra of successive Secretaries of State for Health become 'no investment without reform' (see, for example, Reid 2004), as politicians became concerned about making good use of the additional funds, and expectations about improved performance grew, from both policy-makers and the public.

Central control reorganisation

The programme of changes designed to increase central control and to encourage local NHS organisations to conform to standards and guarantee service improvement were often described in terms of 'delivery' mechanisms, following the establishment of the Prime Minister's Delivery Unit that was responsible for making sure crucial targets were met in public services (Barber, 2007). What they share in common is the attempt to impose a common standard on healthcare delivery, to measure performance against that standard, and to engage in corrective action or reward, depending on their level of achievement. This simple method of exerting control over the delivery of a complex system represents the standard control cycle of cybernetics, or the planning cycle of large corporations, but was very new in the NHS. The actual implementation of the central control programme, however, was rather more complicated than that simple model, and differed considerably in the specifics of its details, depending on the particular part of the health service it was being introduced into.

The NHS Plan required hospitals, providers of primary and community health services and nursing homes to publish an annual prospectus setting out their standards, their performance as it had been measured within the healthcare system and the views of patients. National standards for major health conditions were to be published, with the first National Service Frameworks (NSFs) developed for mental health, coronary heart disease, cancer, older people and diabetes, and with the promise that more would be developed by NICE (and the bodies which succeeded it). The new delivery model proposed that the Department of Health would set standards for care, monitor performance against them, put in place an inspection regime, support the modernisation of health services and correct failures to deliver care. Targets were also set – by 2004, patients were expected to be able to see a primary care professional within 24 hours, and a GP within 48 hours, and 1,000 GPs were to become specialist GPs. Across the NHS, consultants were expected to increase the number of outpatient consultations to four million per year.

The performance management system as outlined in the NHS Plan proposed to put in place a system in which traffic lights would grade the performance of healthcare providers, but in implementation this was (at least initially) turned into a 'star' system, grading performance between zero and three according to a range of performance indicators (DH, 2001c). Sanctions for poor performers were proposed, including the threat that their managerial teams would be replaced and those from high performers would be given control of failing hospitals. Hospitals measured as performing well, in contrast, would be given additional freedoms and the ability to bid for increased funding through a system called 'earned autonomy' (Mannion et al, 2003). Performance ratings were to be published annually.

The highest performing NHS organisations were also encouraged to apply to become foundation trusts, with them being not-for-profit, public corporations accountable to their local communities (who were encouraged to become members). Foundation trusts were meant to be given additional freedoms to manage their affairs, especially in terms of performance management reporting to strategic health authorities, and given the ability to access new sources of financial capital to invest in the development of new services. They were to be overseen by a new independent regulator called Monitor, which could intervene in their affairs in the event of non-compliance with foundation trusts' statutory obligations.

In GP surgeries, the QOF was introduced as a central part of the GMS contract negotiated during the early 2000s, and introduced in 2004. GPs were to measure their achievements against a range of indicators negotiated with the profession, and which were linked back to varying degrees on best practice evidence (Fleetcroft and Cookson, 2006). Points were awarded to individual practices based on the level of achievement made, and four QOF domains were established: clinical (with 80 indicators in 19 clinical areas); organisational (with 36 indicators concerned with clinical records, information for and about patients, clinical and medicines management); patient experience (with five indicators including length of consultation, the result of patient surveys and patient ease of access); and an additional domain (with eight indicators concerned with cervical screening, child health surveillance, maternity services and contraceptive services).

Clinical governance became a statutory duty in which board members of NHS organisations were made responsible for both the clinical and managerial aspects of care (CHI, 2001), integrating responsibilities and attempting to encourage cross-boundary working between clinicians and managers. This led to the generation of 'hybrid' roles that encompassed both managerial and clinical functions (Nio Ong and Schepers, 1998; Freedman, 2002). Further central involvement in the delivery of health services came through the continued work of NICE, which was responsible for assessing whether new drugs and treatments were sufficiently clinically cost-effective to be paid for through NHS funding, and the CHI (and its successors, first the Healthcare Commission and subsequently the CQC), which promised to inspect and investigate organisations that were deemed to be failing in meeting expected performance standards, or where clinical failings had been reported.

The logic of central control

The new delivery model introduced by the NHS Plan gave the Department of Health a clear role in modernising healthcare by setting standards, monitoring performance against them, creating an inspection regime for the NHS and correcting failures in provision. This programme theory of improvement through increased central control was designed to achieve improvements through the use of target setting and the measuring of performance against those targets, with the best performers being rewarded by being given freedoms from performance management regime in the future, but organisations that were measured as performing badly deemed to be failing and being more closely monitored and inspected as a result. The way that central control worked within each of the specific areas outlined above, however, showed differences that can form the basis of a comparison in trying to work out what seems to work best in this type of reorganisation, how it works, where, and for whom.

In terms of the general infrastructure that made central control programmes possible, clinical governance aligned clinical and managerial goals to produce what was meant to be a more coherent managerial structure for care. This, in turn, as the decade went on, fitted within the new quality improvement system in the NHS where national standards were set by NICE. CHI (and the organisations that succeeded in its role) monitored the progress of health organisations towards performance improvement, and local health services were delivered through modernised health services underpinned by clinical governance and professional self-regulation. NHS organisations appointed clinicians to set up and lead clinical governance systems to make quality the centrepiece of care, and to move NHS trusts away from blaming staff for failures and towards, instead, learning from mistakes. In *An organisation with a memory*, Chief Medical Officer Liam Donaldson advocated the need for reporting, organising and analysing information in order to reduce risk for future patients (Donaldson, 2000). The CHI was to inspect every NHS organisation every four years, and any organisation deemed to be low performing more frequently, as well as being sent to inspect organisations where there were more immediate concerns about care quality or patient safety. The CHI was to work closely with the Audit Commission to generate measures for performance assessment, and the NPSA, which was responsible for the reporting and analysis of adverse medical events and near-misses. Finally, the NHS Modernisation Agency was established to try and break down demarcations between professions and to make care more patient-focused and flexible, attempting to help local managers and clinicians redesign local services through programmes of service modernisation using improvement science thinking and concepts. It was designed to 'change the culture' of healthcare – a phrase that was mentioned increasingly frequently into the 2000s and beyond.

The QOF had similar goals to the NHS delivery model introduced in hospitals, in setting clear standards against which GPs could judge their performance through the award of QOF 'points', and thereby increase the quality of their practice against clear targets. This was a direct attempt to change clinical behaviour in GP surgeries, in many respects the hardest place to achieve managerial reach, as it was where doctors had operated on a semi-autonomous basis since the creation of the NHS, and where managerial scrutiny had been almost entirely absent.

In sum, for the first time, a series of institutions were introduced to standardise care and investigate poor performance at the same time as a performance management system was put in place which proposed 'carrots' for good performers and 'sticks' for those measured as being poor. Labour often characterised health policy prior to the 1980s as being based on 'command and control', in contrast to their own 'third way'-based approach (see, for example, the language of the Secretary of State for Health, 1997). However, increased central control over health policy implementation was, if anything, a feature of reorganisation introduced by Labour's reforms following publication of the NHS Plan in 2000.

What the above changes amount to were an outpouring of policy initiatives from Labour in the first half of the 2000s designed to achieve greater central control over the NHS. This was part of Labour's attempt to achieve stronger 'delivery' (Barber, 2007) or implementation of policy, with all government departments becoming more closely monitored and achievements against pre-set targets being reported back to the Prime Minister personally. These systems were intended to make local managers more responsible for the improvement of their services so that public services across the board were modernised to make them more responsive to the needs of their users. As such, the central control programme of changes introduced in the NHS were representative of how other public services were being modernised at the same time, but the sheer scale of change within the NHS perhaps went further than in any other public service. It is therefore important to consider carefully the effects of all this change. What were the outcomes of these top-down changes to the NHS?

Outcomes of the reforms

Research examining the performance management system introduced for NHS trusts around the 'star' system (and its successors) has received a great deal of criticism. McKee (2004) suggested the star system captured only a small part of the work of a healthcare provider, and Goddard et al (1999) that they were being used to identify poorly performing organisations rather than as part of a broader managerial reform to either encourage good performance or identify best practice, placing an emphasis on 'hard' (quantitative measures) to the detriment of 'soft' intelligence as to how well management was performing. Work by Street (2000) found that only small differences in efficiency measures separated high and low performers that were often within the boundaries we might expect from errors in reporting or collection.

However, the strongest criticism of the introduction of the performance management system for NHS trusts was based on the 'gaming' of the measures that they led to. One aspect of this gaming was the link made between the achievement of performance targets and the threat of managers retaining their jobs, so that fear had begun to accompany the process (Hood, 2006). Within the NHS, managers began to refer to those targets against which performance was most closely monitored (which often concerned waiting lists) as 'P45 issues', where failing to achieve them became possible 'sacking offences' and risked them losing their jobs. In the first half of the decade the activities of the Prime Minister's Delivery Unit meant that an 'unprecedented level of prime ministerial attention to public performance data' (Bevan and Hood, 2006b, p 15) was given.

Reported performance in NHS trusts did improve in some areas. There was a decrease in the number of patients waiting 12 months or more for surgical operations (from 40,000 in 2001 to fewer than 10,000 in 2003). Waiting times were reduced almost across the board, showing that making the target so central in managers' thoughts appeared to be having an effect, even if the outcome was not easily disentangled from the increased capacity coming from the government's increased investment in healthcare.

There were increases in the number of patients seen within the four-hour targets by Accident and Emergency (A&E) departments, and Ambulance Trusts increased the number of 'category A' calls (life-threatening emergencies) that were reached within eight minutes between 2000 and 2003. Bevan (2011, p 109) makes clear that he believes that there is 'strong evidence from the evaluations of the star-rating regime that this had a direct and powerful effect in improving the reported performance of the English NHS in terms of shorter hospital waiting times and ambulance response times, both over time, and as compared with the performance of the NHS in the other three countries of the United Kingdom.'

Bevan and Hood (2006b, p 517), however, suggest that there was 'a substantial disparity between reported and actual performance data', highlighting the difficulty in separating the actual performance of trusts with what the measures actually capture, and, in turn, the extent to which they are a function of improved care, or of 'gaming'. Hood (2006) identified three generic gaming effects: ratchet effects, where undemanding targets were put in place by policy-makers with the sole aim of them being easily exceeded; threshold effects, where targets were chosen that gave few incentives for them to be exceeded (such as minimum waiting times); and output distortion or manipulation of expected results, where managers actively changed returns to make their organisations look like they were achieving or exceeding targets when they were not. Bevan and Hood (2006b) suggest there was evidence of gaming of all three types in the NHS, and that organisational returns were being accepted by central government without verification or checking, even where patient survey data contradicted the organisational data being reported by trusts. It was not only academics who were critical of the performance management framework introduced in hospitals. The CHI found evidence of patients having to wait in ambulances before being seen by A&E departments, and beds being created by removing wheels from gurneys to meet A&E waiting targets (CHI, 2003, 2004).

Equally concerning is research that suggested that Ambulance Trusts were increasingly viewing performance indicators as ends in themselves, and that non-measured aspects of their work were becoming neglected as a result, so that paramedics were becoming focused on response times rather than other aspects of their roles, with some stations sending out ambulances without a full complement of fully trained staff in order to reach their destination as quickly as possible (Heath and Radcliffe, 2007). The same study found significant differences between sites in the way that time was measured and emergencies were categorised, again casting doubt on the reliability of the data being used to measure performance.

In terms of public health, achieving reductions in health inequalities was regarded by chief executives as a priority, but in practice was not regarded as being as important as target-focused areas such as waiting times or reaching financial goals (Blackman et al, 2009; Harrington et al, 2009). As the decade wore on, attempts to address health inequalities appeared to be undermined by trying to achieve 'quick wins' through lifestyle and clinical solutions rather than by trying to tackle the more complex and difficult underlying social determinants of health.

And then there were the problems that occurred at Mid Staffordshire Hospital Trust. The Healthcare Commission (one of the successors to CHI) was first called in to investigate reports of high comparative mortality figures in emergency care at the hospital (Healthcare Commission, 2009). The report showed significant clinical failings, with reports of poor performance and complaints not reaching the hospital board. Clinicians believed the trust was driven by financial considerations, and that they were marginalised in decision-making. Perhaps most worryingly, all the agencies created by the government during the 2000s with the specific aim of avoiding trust failure had not noticed the failures or intervened. It was not the routine reporting of Monitor, the Healthcare Commission, the strategic health authority, the PCTs or local government that led to the disclosure of the problems. Equally, it was not picked up by local public and patient forums, with patients' family and friends organising campaigns to expose the care failings at the hospital outside of NHS representative bodies because of their poor experiences of dealing with them.

At the end of the decade, Mid Staffordshire cast a long shadow over the NHS, asking difficult questions with regard to how, given all the work done on performance management systems and clinical governance, such a major failure had been allowed to occur, especially given similar care failings such as those highlighted earlier in the Kennedy Report (Kennedy, 2001). The subsequent Francis Report (Francis, 2013) suggested that a major issue was that the performance indicators the trust was chasing hard to try and achieve foundation trust status had perverse consequences in diverting the attention of managers and clinicians away from patient care. Managers were described as striving to reach targets and to achieve financial balance in order to improve reported performance grading, leading to patients being neglected and clinical staff disengaging from any leadership responsibilities. The Francis Report presents an indictment of how, despite Mid Staffordshire apparently working within a performance management regime that gave a greater degree of central control than had ever been in place in the NHS, the care failure was not effectively communicated to the hospital board, to the care regulators, to other organisations in the NHS that might have been able to intervene, or to the Department of Health. We return to what the case of Mid Staffordshire tells us about NHS care in the 2000s later, but for the moment it is worth making clear the extent to which it suggested that the care failings it documented were due to the inadequate workings of the performance management system.

Performance management in the 2000s

Despite its failings, it is likely that performance management in hospitals led to some improvements that were at least, to some extent, real, but that these improvements were not as significant as reported because of outright fraud in the figures returned, the extent of gaming taking place and the concerns about managers and clinicians becoming excessively focused on hitting targets to the detriment of other aspects of care. It also appeared that longer-term goals, such as those for public health, were ignored for long periods as other, more pressing, targets were chased, and then a range of short-term measures put in place to try and achieve improvements in them rather than systematically attempting to tackle their underlying problems.

As such, in terms of our programme theory, we have identified a range of problems, mostly associated with the extent to which the measures were 'gamed', and whether or not the measures actually capture the reality of hospital performance. We return to these concerns when we reassess the programme theory of central control at the end of the chapter.

Clinical governance

The particular effects of the introduction of clinical governance are hard to assess in themselves as they overlap with so many other initiatives to such a significant extent (a problem more generally with the reorganisations of the 2000s; see Mays and Dixon, 2011; Mays et al, 2011). We can, however, consider evidence that explores how health professionals viewed and experienced its introduction.

Clinical governance and performance management were experienced by clinicians as 'undifferentiated aggregation' (Degeling et al, 2004) which, rather than providing clear, individualised targets and accountability that were relevant to individual practitioners, instead were regarded as being the result of the imposition of externally driven targets about which clinicians had not been consulted (Som, 2005), and which were not relevant to their everyday practice (Chang et al, 2002). The consequence of undifferentiated aggregation was that clinical governance and other central control-based programmes were regarded as being primarily politically motivated measures rather than being based on evidence of what might improve patient care. It seems clinical governance had come some way from being an attempt to get doctors and managers to work more closely together, as it had originally been designed to be.

Important research by Degeling and his collaborators (Degeling et al, 2001, 2003, 2006) suggests that managers and clinicians, rather than coming to common views about the reorganisation based on closer working through clinical governance, instead often had very different perceptions of the reorganisations of the 2000s. This is most clearly illustrated below, in Table 4.1.

Table 4.1: Differing perceptions of aspects of health reforms

	Medical clinicians	Medical managers	General managers
Recognise connections between clinical decision and resources	Oppose	Support	Equivocal
Transparent accountability	Oppose	Support	Support
Systematisation	Oppose	Oppose	Support
Multidisciplinary teams	Oppose	Oppose	Equivocal

Source: Degeling et al (2003, p 651)

Table 4.1 suggests that rather than viewing the aspects of clinical governance in a consensual way, significant differences of perspective existed between different groups based on their particular training and background. These differences have very significant implications in attempts to get the different groups to work better together through initiatives such as clinical governance.

The very different attitudes expressed above risk antagonism emerging between the different professions. Full-time managers appear to try and organise meetings to avoid the input of clinicians or even to exclude them entirely (Forbes et al, 2004; Greener, 2004a, 2005, 2008b), and research from Australia suggests that managers regard clinicians as unstrategic because of their focus on individual patient outcomes rather than outcomes on a larger, organisational scale (Braithwaite and Westbrook, 2004). Medical clinicians, equally, regarded managers as behaving in overtly political ways, being concerned too little with improving decision-making and too much with trying to get their own way (Smith, 2003). Clinicians were often reluctant to share clinical data with managers because they believed that managers would not understand the intricacies involved in its interpretation (Currie and Suhomlinova, 2006).

Hybrid clinical/managerial roles

If clinical governance appeared to show a lack of success in getting different professional groups to work more closely together, an alternative approach was to establish 'hybrid' managerial/clinical roles more widely through the creation of posts such as that of clinical director, with the aim of overcoming barriers to achieving managerial and clinical goals. However, substantial problems also occurred here.

Post-holders in such hybrid roles often found they received little respect or recognition from their clinical peers for taking on such roles (Russell et al, 2010), linking back to earlier research finding that doctors who took on managerial roles struggled to balance their 'part-time' managerial roles with their clinical practice (Fitzgerald, 1994). Instead, doctors tended to regard their managerial roles as being temporary until they returned full time to being a clinician again (Forbes et al, 2004). That doctors regarded the managerial aspects of their work as temporary and part time meant that hybrid post-holders had a strong incentive not to alienate their peers when taking on leadership roles, so making poor clinical practice from their colleagues, where it was found, difficult to challenge (Kitchener, 2000). Hybrid post-holders also found a lack of clarity as to exactly what their role within the organisation was (Buchanan et al, 1997).

Perhaps unsurprisingly, as a result of problems in defining hybrid doctor/manager roles, and of getting doctors to take them on, it is still exceptional for a doctor–manager to have a role at the top level of a trust (Day, 2007). However, doctors do appear to have found ways of drawing on managerial discourses to work more closely with managers, as well as to make themselves better understood by them (Mueller et al, 2003). It may also be the case that the use of managerial vocabularies has made doctors more resource-aware in their decision-making (Llewellyn, 2001).

The research above suggests that there is little evidence of doctors and managers working better together, as they seem to have fundamentally different perspectives on health reorganisations, that hybrid clinical-managers do not feel their roles have been sufficiently clearly defined, that they have not been supported in those roles and that they often regard themselves as only temporary managers and so not wishing to challenge poor clinical practice or to be seen to have crossed over to 'the dark side' and therefore 'lost' to their clinical colleagues. Equally, relations between clinicians and managers, according to the research, still appear to be chiefly characterised by distrust. There have been some gains, with clinicians learning managerial language and acquiring the trappings of managerialism in order to try and communicate better with managers, and becoming more resource-aware in their practices as a result, but some of this may be in order to defend their turf rather than preside over, or enthusiastically embrace changes to their practices (Hunter, 2006). On balance it is hard to see much evidence of improved relations between clinicians and managers or more shared accountability as a result of clinical governance.

Foundation trusts

Under the delivery model introduced in the NHS Plan, foundation trust status was presented as an opportunity for high-performing trusts to gain freedom from the performance management system (Exworthy et al, 2011), being freed from central control and able to become more accountable and responsive to their local communities (Walshe, 2003). Early criticisms of the foundation trust model, however, suggested that they were more likely to suffer from an 'excess of accountability' than the 'earned autonomy' they had been promised, as they would be scrutinised not only by the new independent regulator Monitor, but also by the CHI, local government overview and scrutiny committees and PCTs (Klein, 2003). Hunter (2003, p 213) suggested that the focus and attention given to foundation trusts showed an 'unhealthy preoccupation with acute care' at a time when the government claimed it was developing primary care, and attempting to reduce health inequalities.

Early evidence suggested that foundation trusts were performing no better than other NHS trusts, with waiting time reductions being more or less in line with one another, and that they had demonstrated no major improvements in quality or clinical care (Lewis, 2005), despite the fact that they were a self-selecting group of the highest performing trusts in the NHS.

More recent evidence suggests that foundation trusts tended to perform better than non-foundation trusts, but such differences appear to be long-standing rather than the effect of the introduction of the foundation trust form specifically (Verzulli et al, 2011). In 2008 Monitor reported to the House of Commons Health Select Committee that foundation trusts were performing well financially, with only one receiving a poor rating at that time. Monitor, however, had intervened in five because of poor performance in dealing with the hospital acquired infection MRSA. It reported that governance roles were generally clear, but 16 per cent of the trusts were still not satisfied with their board of directors. The report suggested that there was still a lack of evidence that the foundation trusts had promoted innovation or greater PPI, despite the initial introduction of foundation trusts being justified on the grounds that they would be organisational forms more responsive to their local communities. Allen and Jones suggest (2011, p 27), however, that there is evidence of improved responsiveness, but also accept that foundation trust performance more generally has been rather contradictory, and that 'where there had been a history of poor relationships, these were exacerbated by financial trust status'.

As such, whether or not foundation trust status improved the performance of specific hospitals appears to be strongly related to the specific context of the trust in question – raising questions as to the extent to which policy-makers should be seeking health service improvements through organisational reorganisation when they can appear to be so diversely implemented (see also Dixon and Jones, 2011).

In more general terms, it is hard to cast the foundation trust reforms as a success – they do not appear to have generated improved quality over their non-foundation trust peers, and the evidence of the extent to which they have improved responsiveness or found innovative means of greater community involvement in their activities is equivocal. The one significant area of improvement appears to be in financial management, but even here the improvements have not been universal across all foundation trusts, and it is worth noting the extent to which the Francis Report (Francis, 2013) locates blame for care failure at Mid Staffordshire in the prioritising of achieving financial balance above patient care, an issue that has to be a real concern where systems appear to make financial measures such a priority, especially in the resource-scarce environment the NHS is likely to occupy in the 2010s.

Central control in hospitals: summarising the evidence and adapting the programme theory

To summarise, what we have learned so far from the research in relation to the use of performance management in hospitals is that this reflects a use of central control that sets central targets with little consultation of the staff responsible for implementing them. Staff often perceived the targets as 'undifferentiated aggregation', where little account was taken of the specific context of either particular hospitals or services, and so targets were often regarded as politically motivated rather than being designed to improve care. Different professional groups appear to regard the reorganisations of the 2000s in rather different ways, and clinical governance has not succeeded in getting doctors and managers to work more closely together or been successful in systematising effective hybrid clinical/manager roles. Foundation trusts have had contradictory effects that are often strongly linked to their specific local context, but with little systemic gain. Although targets have led to some improvements, especially in waiting times, it is hard to measure or assess the full extent of these improvements because of widespread gaming. At the same time, the events at Mid Staffordshire indicate that it was possible, despite the increased central control resulting from the new performance management systems, for significant care failure to occur, and to continue to occur and remain unchallenged for a period of several years.

In all, despite some improvements in measured performance in a context of significantly improved NHS funding and staffing numbers as a whole, it is hard to argue that the central control programme of reorganisation appears to have worked well in the hospital setting in that it has led to widespread gaming of the measures and failed to guarantee care quality.

How has the central control programme theory worked in other settings, and what can be learned from them?

Quality and Outcomes Framework

The QOF is the version of the central control programme introduced into GP practices, which are very different care settings from those in hospitals. GPs have a long history as independent contractors with their own regulatory systems, and so represent an extremely challenging context for introducing an attempt at achieving greater central control. What happened as a result of the introduction of the QOF?

First, there appears to have been little opposition to the introduction of the QOF from either GPs or practice nurses (Checkland et al, 2007). There were some concerns that it would lead to an increased workload and reduce the time that could be spent on clinical activities (McDonald et al, 2009a). However, and in contrast to their approach to fundholding in the 1990s, GPs appear to have taken on the extra work associated with the QOF in addition to their care workloads, engaging strongly with it (McDonald et al, 2009a). Understanding why this is gives us key insights into how performance management systems in healthcare can work better.

Evidence of whether GPs experienced increased job satisfaction from these changes is mixed, with some reporting dissatisfaction with what they perceived to be the heavy-handed surveillance associated with the QOF (McDonald et al, 2009a) or the extra workload that has resulted from it (Lovett and Curry, 2007), but others expressing broad satisfaction with its introduction and the new GP contract (Checkland et al, 2008). GPs have certainly taken advantage of the opportunity the new contract offered them to withdraw from out-of-hours work (Spurgeon et al, 2005), even if they are being challenged by the 2010 coalition government to reinstate it. There is even evidence that doctors have become more managerial in their outlook as a result of the introduction of the QOF, being more inclined to challenge the performance of their peers where it is believed they are not engaging with the QOF process (McDonald et al, 2008, 2009a).

Patients seem to be generally happy with the increased monitoring that QOF has introduced, including screening, testing and practice-initiated appointments (Lovett and Curry, 2007; but see also McCartney, 2012, for a different perspetive).

Gaming and the Quality and Outcomes Framework

In contrast with the introduction of central control programmes in hospitals, there seems to be little evidence of gaming in relation to the QOF. GPs appear to have accepted the need to discharge bureaucratic accountability in recording clinical decisions for the QOF (Harrison and Dowswell, 2002) even if this reporting led to increased opportunities for their work to be scrutinised. Some GPs have expressed concern that their care is becoming increasingly checklist or 'tick-box'-driven (Checkland et al, 2007; Hudson 2009), with the most powerful case against the QOF changes being made by McCartney (2012), who suggests that much of the framework is not backed by adequate clinical evidence (a claim also made by Fleetcroft and Cookson, 2006), and that its intrusiveness is interfering with the doctor–patient relationship. In this view, the QOF has led to patients becoming data points rather than individuals (Harrison, 2002), where biomedical information is privileged and GP work routinised (Checkland et al, 2008). However, it is worth emphasising that most research seems to indicate that gaming of the QOF has been minimal, despite these reservations, and so the measured improvements that GPs have shown against the QOF measures seem to be genuine.

Workload associated with the Quality and Outcomes Framework

In addition to GPs taking on extra work, the QOF appears to have resulted in changes in the way workload is managed in surgeries. Some practices have explored substituting other health professionals for doctors as the first point of clinical contact, and others have taken advantage of increased prescribing roles for nurses and allied health professionals to put GPs in a more supervisory role, with their own care being reserved for more complex elements of care (Sheaff, 2009).

A considerable amount of the routine work associated with the QOF has been delegated to nurses and healthcare assistants (Leese, 2007), and there are concerns as to whether sufficient training has been given to meet the challenges of these new roles (McDonald et al, 2009b), even if nurses appear to enjoy the greater autonomy offered (McDonald et al, 2008). Indeed, some nurses regard the QOF as offering them the opportunity to take over the entire function of GP practices in their own right (Sibbald, 2008). At the very least, it seems to have led to increased levels of teamworking between doctors, practice managers and nurses (Lovett and Curry, 2007) – again, a marked contrast with the introduction of central control programmes in hospitals, where closer teamworking does not seem to have occurred, even though there are also some concerns that GPs who used the QOF to take on the status of being specialist practitioners might become isolated from other 'rank and file' doctors (Currie et al, 2009).

The Quality and Outcomes Framework and outcomes

In terms of measurable outcomes, the QOF has been remarkably successful in getting GPs to meet its targets (Edwards and Langley, 2007; Lovett and Curry, 2007), with its system of payment for performance leading to improvements in quality indicators for diabetes (Alshamsan et al, 2010), but it being difficult to disentangle the effects of the introduction of the QOF from other quality initiatives introduced alongside it. It also seems that the introduction of the QOF has done little to address inequalities in age, sex and ethnic groups at practice level (Alshamsan et al, 2010).

Despite the concerns offered above, the QOF has, in terms of achieving its own goals, been a considerable success. Its performance framework is based on specific practices embedded in GP work (McDonald et al, 2007) that doctors have interpreted as being best practice (Maisey et al, 2008). Its introduction was not regarded by doctors as a dramatic change, but instead as one of an incremental series of changes going back to limited list prescribing in the 1980s and the GP contract of the 1990s that emphasised practice nurse involvement and led to the introduction of targets into primary care (Gunstone, 2007). GPs appear to have accepted that a greater outcome focus through the use of performance indicators would lead to a loss of some autonomy (Exworthy et al, 2003). The IT systems introduced to manage the QOF system have embedded new patterns of working into the infrastructure of surgeries, potentially adding to the permanence of the changes (McDonald et al, 2007).

Summarising the evidence on the Quality and Outcomes Framework

It seems that, although some GPs have a negative view of the introduction of the QOF, they generally accept its legitimacy because it is seen as being part of a series of longer-term changes to general practice, and because those delivering it believe that the QOF targets are considered to be based on best practice or clinical evidence. GP practices have responded to the introduction of the QOF by reorganising to meet the QOF's demands, with nurses and other health professionals having the opportunity to take on enhanced roles that those other professional groups appear to enjoy. It is an open question whether the success of GPs in meeting their QOF targets is down to the QOF's linking payment with performance, or whether it is because of GPs believing that the targets they are being asked to meet are embedded in good practice. GPs appear to report the latter: that they have internalised the targets and come to associate them with good practice. Nevertheless, the pay-for-performance element of the reorganisation is also surely significant as well. There remain concerns, however, that the QOF is reducing GP practice to a tick-box approach that interferes in the relationship between doctors and patients, and that the QOF targets themselves are not as evidence-based as GPs often suppose them to be, potentially undermining the legitimacy of the reforms should this view become widespread.

What explains the difference in success between the use of central control programmes in hospitals and general practice?

The research summarised above raises important questions – why is it that central control programmes of reorganisation in hospitals appear to have run into such problems in the form of the gaming of the system, and are regarded as representing the imposition of targets that have little to do with clinical practice? Why has hospital-based performance management led to little innovation in terms of doctors and managers working more closely together, whereas in general practice there seems to have been little or no gaming, and instead practice teams have generally worked together well to achieve the QOF targets?

In hospitals, the central control programme of reorganisation was considered by clinicians and managers to be politically motivated rather than clinically based, and the targets were set at a level of abstraction that meant they were not directly related to everyday clinical practice. There seemed to be a significant disconnect between the often managerial targets and clinical practice, exacerbated by clinicians who take on managerial roles not being well-regarded by their peers and reluctant to challenge poor practice as they believe that, when their 'part-time' managerial role is over, they will be returning to clinical practice and have to work alongside their peers again. In hospital settings there appear to be substantial differences in perspective in the way that managers, doctors and clinical managers regard reforms, making it difficult for clinical governance to work effectively.

The end result of the introduction of performance management in hospitals has often been that targets were regarded as being politically imposed, that doctors and managers were mutually suspicious of one another, making teamwork and trust difficult, with doctors attempting to take on managerial roles struggling in them. This led to the performance management system being extensively 'gamed', making it difficult to separate genuine performance improvement from reported performance gains, but strong grounds for suspecting there are gaps between the two.

In general practice, in contrast, the top-down QOF reforms were generally regarded by practice teams as being based on best practice evidence (even if there are dissenting voices in relation to this point), and the targets set in agreement with the profession at a level that allowed them to be incorporated into everyday clinical practice. Doctors appear to have been prepared to take on the more managerial aspects of managing the QOF, even being prepared to challenge clinical colleagues who do not engage with the process, and to use the QOF as a basis for reconsidering care boundaries and practices within practice care teams. Tasks have been increasingly delegated from doctors to other care professionals, with both doctors and nurses especially being prepared to take on new professional roles, the former as specialist GPs, and the latter as nurse practitioners. The introduction of the QOF appears to have resulted in closer teamworking coming from the use of new roles, and GP practices have been remarkably successful in hitting targets.

A key question is the extent to which the 'pay for performance' nature of the QOF represents a significant motivator for GPs, as this element is not present in the performance management regime in hospitals. GPs themselves, however, appear to regard other factors, such as the ability to organise to meet the challenges of the QOF, and the belief that the QOF represents best practice based on evidence, as more important. This points to GPs regarding intrinsic motivational factors as being more important than extrinsic rewards (Frey and Osterloh, 2002).

Towards a programme theory that can improve central control programmes

What can we learn from the comparison above? It is difficult to disentangle the effects of all the different elements of the two central control programmes, but there are also genuinely important lessons that the two programmes can learn from one another.

Central control programmes work by setting common standards against which performance can be measured, with good or poor performance identified and appropriate action taken. Performance management has a stronger chance of working if the standards and targets are agreed with those who will be responsible for implementing them, and the targets are set at a level that engages with day-to-day practice and that is based on evidence of what works in the service being offered. Those responsible for meeting the targets need to be able to reorganise themselves in teams to allow specialism and tasks to be delegated to the most appropriate member of their team. There is an open question as to whether pay-for-performance might also act a driver of improvement, but the GPs themselves suggest it was not a strong motivator for them conforming to the QOF, and evidence from the business and management literature more generally is equivocal to say the least (Frey and Osterloh, 2012). In short, performance management works better where it is put in place in negotiation with those who are responsible for meeting its targets, and it appeals to their intrinsic motivation, showing they will be adopting best practice or performing care based on the best evidence.

Barriers to better performance management in hospitals

There seem to be five main barriers in taking these performance management lessons from the QOF and introducing better systems into hospitals:

- First, doctors and managers still do not trust one another, and if closer teamworking is going to be achieved, this needs to be addressed.
- Second, doctors, managers and clinical managers appear to have very different perspectives on reforms, and so a greater degree of consensus needs to be achieved among them.
- Third, the targets hospitals are often asked to achieve are at a higher level of abstraction than that of the QOF, and need to be translated into a form that clinicians understand in terms of their everyday practice, and that represent the best clinical evidence in that area.
- Fourth, doctors who take on managerial roles are not held in high regard by their peers who see them as having betrayed their profession or specialty, and as a consequence, find poor clinical practice difficult to challenge.
- Fifth, that it is not only managers who senior doctors distrust, but also one another. Hospital consultants are often unwilling to accept the leadership of doctors from other specialties (Plochg and Klazringa, 2005), leading to the problem that, even if a clinical-managerial hierarchy is put in place, doctors may not feel obliged to conform with it.

So how can these five barriers be overcome?

A starting point is that clinical governance, in order to achieve stronger commitment from clinicians towards its goals, should be delegated down to specialty level, where clinical teams can develop integrated care pathways in which clinical and managerial expertise can be brought together to form teams that combine responsibility for delivering care, but within an environment where autonomy is offered to those teams in terms of exactly how they improve their care pathway (Degeling et al, 2003). This approach has a great deal in common with Total Quality Management (TQM)-based approaches that try and achieve closer teamworking in hospitals (Nwabueze, 2001), the use of clinical microsystems that stress the importance of cross-boundary working to get health professionals and managers to work together better to reach mutually agreed targets (Williams et al, 2009), or the ways in which improving complex issues such as improving patient safety can be tackled (Storey and Buchanan, 2008). Clinical governance needs to be delegated to teams at the speciality level in order to drive service improvement, and to increase accountability.

At the same time, however, hospitals have centrally imposed targets and performance measures that they must meet. To achieve greater buy-in for these targets, there is a crucial role for senior hospital managers to work closely with clinicians to translate the abstract, high-level performance indicators set by the government into low-level, practice-based measures that can be tracked for improvement at the speciality team level. The key difference between the QOF and performance management in hospitals is that the work of setting practice-based targets had already been done by the government – if hospitals are to come to regard their targets as representing evidence-based, practice-led improvements, then senior managers and clinicians need to work together to make sure that they are presented as being part of day-to-day practice using measures that link evidence-based care with higher-level performance measures. If specialty-based clinical teams work together to set their own targets, which will aggregate at a higher level into the improvements the hospital needs to make in order to reach its nationally set performance levels, then the lower-level targets will be meaningful and more achievable. Again, this requires clinical teams to have the ability to reorganise as GP practices have done in order to make the improvements they deem necessary, and for accountability to be genuine.

The issue of whether pay-for-performance could be introduced in some form into hospitals to replicate its use in the QOF is more complex. At a basic level, with many of those working in hospitals still subject to nationally negotiated pay and conditions, this appears problematic, but only if interpreted in the narrowest sense of rewarding teams in specialties through the use of financial payments. However, there are also more intrinsic ways of rewarding high team performance in hospitals through the conspicuous celebration of success, the publication of internal performance data rankings, and even through increased non-pay budgets and so extra resources for the clinical teams that the agreed performance measures appear to suggest are the highest performing.

As with the translation of national performance measures into local clinical targets, this process will need careful negotiation and teamwork between senior managers and clinicians, but there is no reason why it cannot be done. Indeed, in many respects, it is the most central function of management to coordinate their organisation so that everyone within it understands their role through clearly specified targets for teams to achieve (Drucker, 1955).

What all this points to is that successful performance management depends on appealing to the intrinsic motivations of staff. It appeals to their professionalism, giving them a voice in the negotiations over the targets to be met, and makes clear the links between their individual performance and the performance of their organisation as a whole. By making clear the links between individual performance targets and the evidence that underpins them, as well as how individuals are helping meet bigger, organisational goals, staff can be motivated to engage in genuinely local dynamic improvement, being given autonomy in how they meet the targets they have agreed need to be in place. Where targets are regarded as arbitrary and have no links to either evidence or the performance of their organisations as a whole, gaming and other dysfunctional behaviours appear far more likely to occur.

In summary, the success of the QOF offers key messages and lessons for how performance management in hospitals can be more successful. Although the QOF works with smaller clinical teams, more clearly specified, practice-based targets, and offers rewards for the achievement of those targets in ways that the performance measures in hospitals do not, these elements can be translated by senior hospital managers and clinicians into a form where specialty teams can work together more closely to achieve targets they regard as legitimate, and be rewarded by other means for achieving success, rather than the gaming to which they often resort at present.

Improving leadership and teamworking

As well as improving the way that performance management works in hospitals, there is still the need to get clinicians and managers to work more closely together. A key component of this comes through the need for improved leadership development programmes. There is a growing research base in this area that is worth exploring here in depth.

What doesn't work in terms of leadership development

Where development programmes are unsuccessful (as measured by research evaluating them), they do not demonstrate that they have given sufficient attention to the NHS context, instructing clinicians in generic management skills or language without the scope for participants to critique the concepts being used. In these circumstances, clinicians often mobilise against the programmes (Currie, 1998, 1999), dropping out rather the completing them (Currie, 1998), the programmes themselves becoming a focus of conflict between the professional groups they are meant to be bringing together.

Programmes aiming to accredit managers through processes such as the Management Charter Initiative were criticised as being private sector-based and so unable to take account of the specific health service and public sector context (Holman and Hall, 1996; Reedy and Learmonth, 2000). Clinicians often regard effective leadership to be embedded in their specific work context (Jahrami et al, 2009), and so generic, competency-based management development approaches are likely to be perceived as being separate from their practice, and therefore of little use.

Development programmes that ignore or do not adequately deal with the different perspectives clinicians and non-clinical managers bring to their roles also often struggle to succeed. There is a danger of professional identities clashing with the managerial perspective that courses tend to present, with one particular NHS-led development programme being singled out for failing to deal with this conflict (Currie, 1996, p 10). In that programme clinical participants suggested that delivery consisted of 'buzzwords'.

There are dangers of misunderstandings because of the different approaches to research and evidence in clinical and managerial practice. The idea of evidence-based medicine has been central to practice since at least the 1990s (Muir Gray, 1996), whereas the application of evidence to management practice is still rather uneven and in its early days (Walshe and Rundall, 2001), and faces considerable (or perhaps even insurmountable) difficulties because of the complexity of the phenomena it must investigate (Learmonth and Harding, 2006). Treating evidence as an idea that applies universal standards of proof to all kinds of research is therefore likely to lead to mutual incomprehension between professional groupings. Clinical participants trained in critical evidence formulation often find the lack of opportunity to engage critically with the generic management concepts presented during management development programmes frustrating, and so they either leave early or reject them as a result. Development programmes that pay insufficient attention to the NHS context are poorly received, and research concerning them emphasises that 'sensitivity to context is important' (Currie, 1999, p 58).

Managers and clinicians may also be suspicious of one another because of their different educational backgrounds and different expectations of personal development. Clinicians are required to engage with continuing education throughout their careers, but managers may often not face the same demands or have the same opportunities (Davies, 2006). Managers may therefore be less familiar with training processes than clinicians, and so be less used to their format and processes.

From the brief synthesis above of the success or otherwise of development programmes, we are able to develop an emergent theory of what is not perceived as effective in management development programmes between clinicians and managers. Because clinicians and managers (and those with a role that encompasses both perspectives) often have different views on the organisational challenges that they face, they are likely to reject development programmes. This is also likely to happen where programmes attempt to induct clinicians uncritically into management ideas, especially where such ideas are not rooted in the kinds of challenges and problems that clinicians can engage with, or where the justification for a practice does not reflect different understandings of research and evidence that exists between clinical and managerial settings. Problems are especially likely to occur where management training practices appear to be derived from private industry contexts. Clinicians are trained to scrutinise evidence grounded in very specific approaches to research that may not be possible to reproduce or replicate when considering the open, complex systems that managerial research is often engaged with, needing programmes to discuss the different approaches to research and evidence they entail. If these differences are not explored, there is a danger of training programmes being challenged by clinicians as being based on inadequate evidence, and of managers becoming frustrated by clinicians' constant challenge of their practices.

In sum, leadership development programmes that attempt to bring clinicians into the managerial world are likely be alienating for clinicians who find management concepts inadequate in explaining the challenges they face, and reject its theory as not based on evidence of a kind they have been trained to value.

What is perceived to be more effective in leadership development programmes

Now that we have worked out what does not appear to be well received by leadership development participants, we are in a position to begin to consider what might be a more successful approach to getting clinicians and managers to work better together.

The leadership development programmes that respondents and researchers evaluate as successful tend to share particular characteristics. Programmes that give clinicians a background in managerial concepts but allow them to engage more successfully with managers across a wider range of organisational issues not rooted in uncritical, acontextual understandings of management, tend to be more successful. This relates back to the issue raised above – where managerial ideas are treated in a sloganistic way, without critical reflection, they are likely to be judged as having little intrinsic value by clinicians, and especially by doctors (Currie, 1996).

Development programmes run in the North West (Allen, 1995) and North East (Carr et al, 2009) have made progress towards these goals, with the North East's particular success being attributed to allowing individuals time to reflect on their practice. In Trent early career doctors and managers were brought together to consider live issues in their organisation as well as using simulation and role-play that was linked explicitly to practice (Owen and Phillips, 2000). This approach was considered to have worked well in facilitating mutual understanding between clinicians and managers. In Dorset, general practices have been successfully supported through half-day development events held away from the workplace to become familiar with management concepts but, more significantly, through programmes that were based on practical problem-solving and that stressed interprofessional collaboration (Headrick et al, 1998).

As noted above, understandings of evidence differ between clinicians and managers from non-clinical backgrounds and this has the potential to be a source of conflict. However, opportunities to critically explore these differences also offer the potential to develop greater appreciation of different perspectives, especially if the reasons for those differences can be discussed openly (Davies, 2006). The design also has to allow flexibility, with participants valuing responsiveness to participant feedback during the programme and allowing for particular issues of concern to the participants to be prioritised (Carr et al, 2009).

There are differences of opinion as to whether development programmes should bring together actual interprofessional work teams to focus on a specific problem they are encountering (Williams et al, 2009), or whether working with clinicians and managers from other NHS organisations is more effective in that it prevents the problem from overwhelming the appreciation of different professional perspectives (Carr et al, 2009). In either case, however, the emphasis on developing practice-led models of training, addressing problems interprofessionally, and a strong awareness of the NHS organisational context appear to be the main factors to the event being successful.

The successful factors above have a great deal in common with the approach to development recommended through a 'deliberate practice' understanding (Anders, 2009) which similarly places an emphasis on understanding organisational contexts and training design that is based on practical problem-solving within those specific domains (Colvin, 2008). Management knowledge, in such a view, is based more on practical problem-solving, often facilitated through in-depth case studies (Griseri, 2002) than on the teaching of generic competencies.

This research review points to a programme theory that more accurately reflects what is perceived to be successful about NHS leadership development. The context of NHS organisational development is one where different professionals, often with very different views of the world, need to learn to work together better. Leadership development interventions should therefore be designed with the aim of getting both clinical and managerial teams from particular settings together to learn and solve problems alongside one another. Working with professionals from different backgrounds to better understand the policy context is a viable strategy that can add to shared understandings, can often be a means of both showing that development programmes will be relevant to them, and provide a shared framework within which learning can take place. Leadership development programmes should not be based on generic management frameworks that are assumed to be equally relevant in both private and public sectors, but rooted in specific challenges and problem-solving that the professional groups need to solve together. The use of case-based methods can be a viable strategy, making use of adapted materials such as those provided in detailed empirical case studies from funders such as the National Institute for Health Research, and aiming to generate multiprofessional understandings of the problems NHS organisations face in order to foster an environment of more mutual understanding.

In short, what works for leadership development is for multidisciplinary health teams to have the opportunity to train together, utilising problem-driven material that takes account of the specific context of healthcare in order to help clinicians and managers to better understand that context, and to appreciate and critically interrogate the different perspectives they can bring to solve problems of the type they will have to face at work.

Supporting health managers and clinicians to work together better

Given the discussion above, a number of propositions can be put forward as to the best means of supporting health managers and clinicians in the specific context of healthcare, especially in relation to the previous two chapters:

- Hybrid clinical/managerial roles in particular need much stronger support from both clinicians and non-clinical managers in order to achieve the demanding goals required of clinical leadership. The problem-based, collaborative design approach advocated here is one way of such support being provided, but organisational design needs to ensure that both doctor-manager and nurse-manager roles are given the authority and status they deserve in NHS management.
- NHS leadership development needs to be organised on a problem-based, multiprofessional collaborative basis to ensure that clinicians are not isolated by being taught generic management theory, and that all participants are able to contribute their professional expertise to practical, problem-solving tasks that will inform their teamworking in real life situations. An additional advantage is that, with careful facilitation, different professional groupings can gain insights into the differing evidence bases of clinical and managerial research, and learn to respect work of each type and their potential contribution to understanding and overcoming the challenges faced in everyday practice.
- Case-based material represents a pedagogical tool that is likely to facilitate greater collaboration and closer teamworking through the use of practical problem-solving it can achieve. The UK National Institute for Health Research, and in particular its Health Services and Delivery Research funding programme, for example, now has an extensive library of such material that might form the basis of content used in development programmes, as well as increasing the take-up of its funded research, and using previous research in this way represents a significant opportunity.

It is perhaps not surprising that NHS leadership development, in common with management development in other settings in the private and public sectors, conducts little research into the long-term return on investment of such programmes or the difficulties in transferring learning into the workplace. These remain difficult research questions in the field of leadership development more generally and, as ever, will require considerable investment and longitudinal studies to assess whether training is meeting the needs of health organisations rather than meeting the expectations of its participants.

Conclusion

This chapter has covered a great deal of ground in considering the use of central control programmes of reorganisation in the 2000s. It has contrasted especially the introduction of such programmes in hospitals and GP surgeries, and suggested that we can present a revised theory of how central control programmes can work better, not only in healthcare, but in public services more generally.

To reiterate, central control programmes work by setting common standards against which performance can be measured, with good or poor performance identified, and appropriate action taken. They appear to have a better chance of working well if the standards and targets to be used are agreed with those who will be held responsible for their implementation, if the targets are at a level that is engaged with day-to-day practice, and where those responsible for implementing them regard the targets as being based on evidence or best practice. Finally, those who are responsible for implementation need the ability to reorganise themselves in teams to allow for specialisation and for tasks to be allocated to appropriate team members. These factors all point to the need for performance management to engage with the intrinsic motivations of staff – of showing them that they should achieve targets because it means that they will be doing a good job in terms of patient care. Whether pay-for-performance would improve such a system remains an open question, but does run counter to the intrinsic satisfaction argument that the other factors appear to rest on.

In terms of overcoming the barriers between clinicians, leadership development training offers some answers. In such training it is crucial that the specific contextual factors present in healthcare are taken into account. Such programmes are more likely to work better where multidisciplinary health teams have the opportunity to train together, with such training utilising problem-driven material that takes full account of the specific context of healthcare and which allows teams to better understand that context, and to appreciate and critically interrogate the different perspectives they can bring to solve problems of the type they will have to face at work.

Having considered central control programmes or reorganisation in the 2000s, and made modifications to the programme theory to suggest performance management and clinical governance systems can be improved in hospitals in particular, the book now moves to consider the attempts at 'dynamic local' programmes of reorganisation during the same decade. What does the evidence tells us happened as a result of the extension of patient choice, the reintroduction of the market for care, and the repeated reorganisation of patient and public consultative arrangements in the 2000s?

FIVE

Local dynamic reform in the NHS since 2000

Introduction

For much of the history of the NHS, individual hospitals, GP surgeries and community health providers have been only indirectly linked to the Department of Health. The government has set the budget of the NHS, and put in place new organisational structures (as it did in 1974 and 1990), but for the most part, the day-to-day activities of most health organisations have been remarkably insulated from the control of influence of the organisational tiers above them, or from government itself. The previous chapter explored how this changed during the 2000s, when a performance management system was put in place that imposed a great deal more central control on both hospitals and GP practices, to varying degrees of success. This chapter explores how policy-makers attempted to get health organisations to improve by putting in place what we have called 'local dynamic' mechanisms to attempt to drive improvements.

'Local dynamic' mechanisms differ from central control reform mechanisms in that, although they are imposed centrally by government, they attempt to create locally based dynamics that may vary in operation from context to context, but that seek to generate improvement in a self-sustaining way. Central control mechanisms such as performance management require a central department to put in place incentives to improve by monitoring the activities of organisations, measuring them, and responding appropriately by either rewarding good performance or penalising bad. Local dynamic mechanisms, in contrast, attempt to generate mechanisms by which organisations can become self-improving, and so do not need the continual intervention of a central department.

The two mechanisms are summarised below, in Table 5.1.

Chronologies of health policy during the 2000s, and indeed the accounts of government advisers (Warner, 2011), suggest that the early part of the decade was dominated by central control measures, after which a more concerted attempt was made to introduce local dynamic mechanisms (often alongside the central controls) (Greener,

Table 5.1: Central control and local dynamic mechanism

	Central control	Local dynamic
Means of improvement	Setting and achieving standards	Competition Input from patient groups
Benchmark/gauge of success	Central standard as fixed measure	Maintenance of existing contracts Gaining new contracts Patient and public approval
Carrot	Foundation trust status 'Earned autonomy' Intrinsic motivation	More resources (PbR) Improvements leading to less regulatory interference
Stick	Franchisement of management Naming and shaming	Loss of contracts Complaints from patients and public Regulatory interference if care does not improve
Standards	Centrally set (may be locally tailored to fit central standards)	Made in comparison with local competition (hospitals), or against local expectations (public)

2004b; Stevens, 2004). The director of the Prime Minister's Delivery Unit suggested that by the mid-2000s top-down performance management systems (central control) were running up against their limits, and further improvements needed a new, bottom–up philosophy of improvement instead (local dynamic) (Barber, 2007). Even if we treat this narrative of reorganisation from the government as something of a post-hoc rationalisation to try and justify shifting power or accountability from the centre to the localities, and which conceals central control mechanisms continuing to operate alongside local dynamic attempts at change, treating the two types of reorganisation as separate programme theories gives us a means of attempting to assess their effects independent of one another.

Both central control and local dynamic mechanisms existed in the NHS prior to the 2000s. The internal market of the 1990s can be regarded as an attempt to get healthcare providers to compete with one another to generate improvements, and the introduction of community health councils in the 1970s were meant to introduce a stronger voice for patients in improving their local health services, so both utilised local dynamic mechanism. In the second half of the 2000s, however, the government became committed to the reintroduction of market mechanisms alongside repeated reorganisations of PPI organisations, generating a distinctive local dynamic programme theory for the generation of self-sustaining improvement.

This chapter reviews research on the introduction of patient choice and competition (alongside the introduction of PbR) and the reorganisation of PPI systems within the NHS. These were both designed to create self-sustaining systems of improvement, the first by introducing a competition-based dynamic designed to drive up service responsiveness and clinical quality, and the second by encouraging 'voice' mechanisms by which patients and the public could be more involved in the governance of health service organisations to become more patient-focused. We begin by reviewing the research on patient choice and the reintroduction of competition into the NHS.

Patient choice and competition

As noted in earlier chapters, the idea of introducing competition between healthcare providers in the NHS is not a new one. In the 1990s the government introduced a quasi or internal market to secure precisely those ends. During that decade, providers of care were separated from purchasers, with providers being expected to compete for contracts from local authorities and GP fundholders who were given budgets to purchase care on behalf of their patients. However, there was not much of a market for healthcare in the 1990s (West, 1998), with competition limited in that it overwhelmingly involved public providers only, and most hospital referrals went to areas local to patients (Exworthy and Peckham, 2006). In GP fundholding practices, often regarded as the most dynamic element in the reforms (Robinson and Le Grand, 1994; Goodwin, 1998), healthcare decisions were made by doctors on behalf of their patients rather than by the patients themselves (Greener and Mannion, 2006, 2009a), and doctors appeared reluctant to refer patients to new providers, even in those cases where patients were willing to travel to them (Exworthy and Peckham, 2006). Labour, on coming to power in 1997, claimed to have abolished the internal market on the grounds it was bureaucratic and wasteful (Secretary of State for Health, 1997; although see also Powell, 1998).

After 2000, however, the government appeared to have become interested in the use of market mechanisms in the NHS again. In 2001, a discussion document suggested that patients should be offered increased choice (DH, 2001b) as a means of driving improvements in healthcare, and a pilot project was set up in London to explore whether those waiting for more than six months for their care referral could be persuaded to move to an alternative hospital for their care.

Despite the tendency of both academics (see, for example, Le Grand, 2007) and policy-makers to present the London pilot on patient choice as supporting the extension of patient choice nationally, its form in London was very different from the way choice-based reorganisations was implemented in the rest of the country. In the London pilot patient choice was supported through advisers and paid-for transport, and was largely concerned with offering patients who had waited a long time the choice of going to an alternative provider which could see them more quickly. Patient choice in the rest of the country was about every patient being referred from GP surgeries being offered a choice of providers, but without the support of patient choice advisers, and usually without any support for transportation. Even the government acknowledged how important patient choice advisers were for the policy (Office of Public Services Reform, 2005), and so their omission from the implementation in the rest of the country seems significant.

The 'mixed economy of care' appeared during the 2000s through a series of gradual changes, and it was not until the second half of the decade that all the components were in place based on four elements: patient choice, provider diversity, PbR and quality and financial regulation (Dixon and Jones, 2011, p 114). The consultative document on extending patient choice (DH, 2001b) was followed by the introduction of PbR (DH, 2002; Dixon 2004), which attempted to try and achieve the goal of money following patient referrals, so that attractive providers received the most resources. At the same time, the government attempted to extend competition by encouraging entry from non-public providers into the NHS through the strategic use of the 'tariff', or fixed price for care, to encourage more non-public provision so that, by 2011, the private sector in England received 25 per cent of its revenue from the public purse (McLellan, 2012).

By 2006, the government put in place a guarantee that patients would be offered a choice of at least four providers for their secondary referrals, facilitated by the introduction of an IT system called Choose and Book that allowed appointments to be made direct from either GP surgeries or via the telephone later.

The patient choice and competition reforms were to be based on a fixed-price for care system (the 'tariff'), as opposed to purchasers and providers negotiating contracts in the 1990s, that was intended to encourage providers to focus on quality rather than to compete on price. Equally, there was an increased emphasis on patients making choices concerning the provider to whom they would be referred rather than relying on their GPs, with the NHS Choices website being set up and providers of care encouraged to provide information leaflets about their services on which such choices could be based. Such information, however, was often limited to presenting the government's performance management statistics in a more accessible form, and information was not disaggregated to service level (see, for example, Easington PCT, 2006).

The local dynamic programme theory of choice and competition was an attempt to try and achieve self-sustaining improvement by introducing a dynamic of competition into local health areas in which providers of care would compete with one another to receive contracts and care referrals, with PbR moving resources to the providers who were most successful in attracting them. The resulting competitive dynamic would drive up care standards. What was the effect of these changes?

Research on patient choice and competition

Patient choice and competition reorganisations in both the 1990s and 2000s place an emphasis on GP practices being where doctors and patients can discuss treatment options in an informed and open way, coming to decisions about referrals together or by patients leading the choice process to ensure their wishes are met, with GPs regarded as the clinical professionals most able to understand their patients' needs.

Research examining doctor–patient relations in surgeries, however, presents a picture that questions whether GPs are best-placed to act on behalf of their patients. The short duration of GP consultations makes including patients in referral decisions difficult, especially for more vulnerable patients who need additional support. Equally, the Choose and Book computer system designed to support choice has often not worked well (Weir et al, 2007). GPs often have little time or scope in their consultations for patients to make choices (Bryan et al, 2006), and even where patients believe they are being consulted by doctors, independent observers of consultations find that around three quarters of decisions made in GP practices are predominantly by doctors (Ford et al, 2006). There is evidence that GPs treat patients differently depending on how attractive they perceive them to be (O'Reilly et al, 2006), being prepared to spend more time and engage in more interaction with the patients they prefer. There are also questions as to which health professional is best placed to provide referral choice advice to patients, with research asking significant questions as to whether GPs have the critical interpersonal skills to support patient choice (Ford et al, 2006).

In addition, GPs were found to be reluctant to use electronic booking because of technical issues, not being able to refer to a named consultant, increased consultation times, lack of appointment slots and inaccurate and inconsistent information (Dixon et al, 2010b). Referral patterns were considered stable by providers, rather than being driven by quality, and leading to providers competing for GP referrals rather than patients. The independent sector was rarely a threat to the public sector, acting instead as a partner supplying extra capacity.

Where patients are unhappy with their GPs, the local dynamic approach was meant to make it easier for them to move to another practice. This may be the case theoretically, but in practice patients remain extremely loyal to their GPs, usually only changing them in situations of significant disaffection (Robertson et al, 2008). This does not necessarily mean, however, that patients are happy with the service GPs provide. Rather, such loyalty may be down to inertia, or the belief that changing practice will take up time patients do not feel they have. Indeed, research shows that the choice of GP practice is more often a function of picking the practice closest to home rather than making a meaningful decision based on care quality (Greener, 2003).

If we were to restructure GP appointments to allow choice to be meaningfully explored, it would seem to require a dramatic change in the way that such consultations are conducted; they would need to be longer, and require GPs to be more sensitive about how their own biases may be affecting their care decisions, as well as requiring GPs themselves to acquire a far stronger knowledge of their local health areas to provide evidence-based advice about referrals.

Given the lack of time in GP consultations for patients to make referral decisions, a common strategy has been for telephone-based systems to be used. Patients, after their consultation, are then asked to ring a telephone number to book their appointment, but it is hard to see how patients can be making informed decisions about where they are to be referred without access to comparative information concerning possible providers of care (Appleby and Dixon, 2004). It was a central message of the London patient choice pilot that the quality of the support given to patients when making a choice was crucial (Rossiter and Williams, 2005).

When these findings are combined, it suggests overwhelmingly that it is doctors who make decisions about referrals in GP surgeries, and that patients are not being treated equally. If increasing patient choice is important for local dynamic reorganisation, then it is not clear how it can be accomplished with GP practices working in this way.

The Department of Health found in 2009 that only 50 per cent of patients remember being offered a choice of referral providers by their GPs, and that only a tiny proportion had made use of the NHS Choices website (Dixon, 2009). Few patients appear to have consulted any kind of published information at all (Marshall and McLoughlin,

2010) in making choices, with them depending instead on 'personal experience, the advice of trusted professionals (usually the GP) and the reputation of a hospital' (Dixon and Robertson, 2011, p 63). The King's Fund found that the evidence on patient choice suggests 'that policy-makers should not rely on patients alone to drive quality improvement' (Dixon and Robertson, 2011, p 65).

Research examining secondary care since the introduction of patient choice suggests that referral patterns from primary care are often based more on historical precedent than the careful assessment of evidence by GPs. Even where particular providers have experienced widely reported adverse clinical events, GPs continue to refer to them, and patients appear to be loyal to those services where they have already experienced them (Greener and Mannion, 2009a). More widely, where there have been high-profile investigations into particular providers over patient safety, it seems that patients continue to choose them (Laverty et al, 2012). If increased patient choice is meant to be driving improvements in care quality, then GPs continuing to refer to services that have been shown to have problems, and patients continuing to choose them regardless, seems to be a significant barrier to achieving this end.

There is evidence, however, of patient choice working in some limited contexts. The King's Fund suggests that in rural locations, 'where no single provider dominated and people were more used to travelling to access services' (Dixon and Robertson, 2011, p 65), there was greater scope for its approach working, but even then it seems likely that older, highly educated people with their own transport were more likely to embrace patient choice (Dixon et al, 2010b), suggesting it could be source of inequality.

Patient choice and the Quality and Outcomes Framework

We noted in Chapter Four that the QOF has been remarkably successful in achieving the goals set for it, leading to reorganisations of GP practices to achieve the targets set within it. However, as the QOF is explicitly meant to represent targets based on clinical evidence, and as the evidence-based movement has generally led to the use of guideline-driven care more extensively, this often conflicts with offering patients choices about their treatment (Rogers, 2002). McCartney (2012) describes how, because of the QOF and the increased use of guideline and protocol-driven care, she finds herself continually confronted by computer-initiated prompts in relation to the patients she finds before her in the GP practice, having less time and scope for actually talking and finding out the root cause of the difficulties they bring to her.

Equally, as noted in Chapter Three, there is a trend towards GPs acquiring special interests, and in reorganising their practices so that they see patients who would formerly have been referred to consultants in secondary care. However, research suggests that patients prefer to be seen by hospital consultants ('specialists') where they believe their care is above the level they associate with their GP practice, and are more tolerant of poor treatment from consultants than they are from GPSIs performing the same care (Horrocks and Coast, 2007). Patients who experience care from GPSIs are often happy to receive care from them again, but given a choice of provider (including their GP), they prefer to be seen by consultants. There are tensions between the care patients should receive according to clinical evidence, and the choices patients might want to make themselves. These are illustrated by the presence on every high street of alternative medicine practitioners (such as Chinese medicine), and of the huge growth in popularity of complementary and alternative medicine in the last two decades more generally, when few of these treatments (if any) are supported by any robust (as it is conceptualised in the evidence-based medicine movement) evidence. If health policy is increasingly placing patient choice at its centre, then conflicts between clinical evidence and the treatments patients want, regardless of that evidence, are set to come to the fore.

Information and patient choice

Since 2006 governments have continually suggested that if patients receive better information, they will make better healthcare referral choices. The research presented above seems to cast some doubt on this. Why should this be the case? Surely we all want to receive the best possible care? One explanation for this comes in studies of tools designed to support patients in making care choices that find that they do not have any effect in reducing patients' anxiety over treatment or in improving their satisfaction with the care decisions that they make (O'Connor et al, 2009). Improving referrals is not just about providing more information to patients – they may actively prefer doctors to make decisions on their behalf (Ford et al, 2006), and feel uncomfortable where they do not regard themselves to be qualified to make a complex decision about their care. Patients do not so much want choice as a good service where they are consulted about treatment and listened to (Curtice and Heath, 2012, p 500).

The problems of patient choice are further exacerbated by patients saying prospectively (before they are ill) that they would like a greater say in their care and treatment, but in situations where they have serious illnesses, such as cancer, preferring doctors to make decisions on their behalf (Schwartz, 2004). Experimental studies in a range of health areas where patients face difficult choices with potentially adverse physical or psychological consequences suggest they simply do not want to have to face those choices (Iyengar, 2010). The assumption that patients want choices about their care decisions, or are equipped to make them, is not supported by these studies, regardless of opinion poll data in which the public may say that they want greater choice.

Finally, a National Institute for Health Research synthesis of research on patient choice conducted in the mid-2000s, when patient choice policies were being rolled out in England, suggested that very few patients actually want to choose the healthcare provider to which their GP refers them, instead preferring an assurance that they are to receive good quality care from a local health service (Fotaki et al, 2005). How far patients are prepared to travel in order to receive better care, and whether the costs this imposes on them are reasonable, remain live issues within the debate around patient choice.

Econometric research on patient choice

The research presented above suggests that the policy from successive governments to extend patient choice might be misconceived. Despite opinion poll data saying that the public want increased choices over their health services, GPs continue to make most care decisions, patients experience considerable anxiety over making choices where they involve what they regard as important decisions, they do not use tools such as the NHS Choices website designed to support their choice, and when they do use such tools, they find they do not improve their satisfaction with the decisions that they make. Referral decisions made in GP surgeries appear to be based on historical referral patterns rather than on careful evaluation of who the best provider of care might be, even where particular providers have had significant clinical safety problems. In short, the policy of extending patient choice seems to have little potential to improve clinical care.

There is, however, research that suggests that the introduction of patient choice post-2006 has had a range of positive effects in secondary care. This work, as it appears to contradict the research above, therefore needs careful assessment. Gaynor et al (2010, 2012) suggest that the changes post-2006, after which patients were offered a choice of providers for secondary referrals, and where PbR was in place so that resources followed from their choices, has meant the introduction of competition into the NHS in England. They suggest that this has led to changes in travel patterns for patients in and around conurbations, so that, according to their measure, hospitals with shorter waiting lists and higher clinical quality received more referrals. Cooper et al (2011) found that hospitals that, according to their measure, face more competition, had both a bigger improvement in clinical quality after 2006 than those that faced less competition, as well as shorter lengths of stay. The findings from the last team have been summarised in publicity arising from their work, claiming that 'competition saves lives', and was cited in the 2010 coalition White Paper on NHS reform (Secretary of State for Health, 2010) as supporting an extension of competition mechanisms in healthcare.

This econometric research, which claims to have found positive benefits from the extension of patient choice post-2006 despite concerns expressed in the detailed empirical studies of GP practices cited above (although it does not cite or engage with this work, so the researchers are perhaps unaware of it), therefore makes strong claims about how well it has worked. It suggests that the use of patient choice has led to a significant change in referral patterns towards hospitals with shorter waiting times and higher clinical quality, and that hospitals in the most competitive areas have experienced the biggest improvements in clinical quality and lengths of stay. How can it be that this work produces such different results from the work presented earlier in the chapter?

A first point to make is that the work cited earlier is based on empirical observation of patients and doctors in different healthcare settings, whereas the econometric work is, instead, based on a 'black box' method (Bevan and Skellern, 2011) that attempts to use quantitative data to find relationships between variables through the use of controls, and to establish causation on those grounds. The King's Fund's evaluation suggested it is 'weak with regard to exactly how competition between hospitals for elective patients might result in the staff (particularly the clinical staff) improving quality of care in non-elective areas such as myocardial infarction' (Propper and Dixon, 2011, p 87). The econometric research is dependent on showing that the post-2006 NHS has seen the introduction of a market for care, and that healthcare providers and patients responded to the changed incentives that were introduced at that point (Mays, 2011). However, these changes are assumed in the research rather than being empirically investigated – and the findings from studies cited above suggest that clinicians and patients were not behaving significantly differently post-

2006. Patients were not using the NHS Choices website to make the kind of informed choices the econometric work would appear to require (Dixon and Wright, 2008), and GPs lacked the information to make such changes. Equally, even if hospitals were now facing a regime in which payments for care followed patient choice, it is less clear that individual consultants had an incentive to improve their care – it would be historically remarkable if doctors were to be sacked because their organisation faced financial difficulties of any kind, and everything we know about the NHS since its inception highlights the scale of the challenge involved in getting managers, who might be threatened by their organisation facing a financial deficit, to change clinical behaviour.

Equally, the econometric research does not demonstrate that competition was actually taking place – it assumes that if there are more hospitals within a particular travel time or distance from a GP practice, then there will be a more competitive environment. This may or may not be an accurate assumption, and needs careful additional research. Additional providers might create as much an incentive for collaboration as competition.

What Gaynor and Cooper's research shows is that there has been a range of important changes in referral patterns and clinical outcomes since 2006, but this was at a time, as Chapter Four makes clear, when a raft of health reforms were being implemented. We simply cannot specify outcomes to particular reforms when such large-scale, systemic reform was taking place simultaneously. We need close empirical research and a large-scale evaluation of patient choice and competition reforms in order to assess their impact. Claiming that they have achieved such improved clinical outcomes without even being able to show that competition existed, or without being able to explain exactly how the effects were meant to have happened (except by claiming it was due to competition), appears premature to say the least, especially when that work has been used so explicitly by the government to justify further reform (Greener, 2012).

What kind of choices do patients want?

From the evidence presented so far, it would seem sensible to conclude that most patients don't seem to particularly want increased choice over referrals. But this is a very narrow definition of patient choice – do patients want other kinds of choices?

When being asked to make a choice about care referral, many patients find the choice of possible providers confusing, especially as they often have little time to make their decision, and because the tools designed to help support their decision do not reassure them or improve their decision. Patients do, however, want to enter into a collaborative relationship with clinicians to make decisions about their care (Rozmovits et al, 2004), and where patients have long-term conditions, the scope increases for patients to become more informed, not only about the provision of care in their local area, but also about their clinical condition. In such circumstances, they can take on greater responsibility for their care, should they wish to, and become an 'expert patient' (DH, 2001a). Where patients are able to become self-managing in this way, it is clearly of benefit to both doctors and patients for them to do so. It is easy to imagine a situation, were the NHS ever to put in place comprehensive information systems linked to patient records, that there is huge scope for patients to engage more pro-actively with care choices and to be far more aware of their own health histories (Taylor, 2012), but this is still some way off.

For the moment, the kind of choice most patients would like when being referred to a secondary provider is not *which* provider they should be referred to, but *when* they are to be seen. Ideally, we would all like to be referred at a time and to a place of our choosing, and this is likely to mean receiving care close to where we live at a time that suits us.

There are substantial barriers to offering this kind of patient choice, however. Choose and Book, the information system that underpins health reform, is not structured to achieve this end as it is primarily based on offering a choice of different providers rather than finding a provider who can offer care at a suitable time.

Indeed, where waiting lists exist, it may be neither efficient nor equitable for patients to be able to choose exactly when they will be seen as this will remove any discretion doctors are able to exert about how urgent one person's needs are in relation to another's, and could lead to the possibility of the most clinically urgent patients having to wait while less urgent cases are seen first. This does not seem entirely fair or even an effective use of resources.

As such, patient choice is most likely to work in long-term conditions where patients have the time and motivation to gain knowledge of their condition, and are able to work with clinicians, preferably through established relationships. In such a situation patients will be able to exercise genuine choice over medication, treatment and which provider treats them in an informed way. For many other care decisions, however, extending patient choice has significant problems in that it has tended to focus on offering a choice of referral provider – which may be the choice most patients value least – instead of when patients will be treated – which raises equity and efficiency issues. In either case, patients are not making much use of the government-sponsored websites designed to provide them with information about their care referrals (Ramesh, 2010).

Partnership working and competition

If the 2000s saw the widespread use of performance management and the reinstatement of competition, there was also a considerable emphasis on partnership working. At first sight, this appears to represent something of a contradiction. At the same time as individual hospitals and GP services were being more strongly performance-managed than ever before, and providers were being asked to compete with one another and purchasers to choose between them, health service organisations were being asked to engage in partnership working with one another, as well as engaging in closer partnerships with social care organisations. It is to state the obvious that people's needs to not always correspond to service boundaries, and it is often the people with the most complex needs – who are themselves often the most vulnerable – who require partnership working the most.

There are certainly conflicts between partnership working and competition, and if the unit of assessment for performance management is the individual unit (hospital, GP practice) rather than the whole local health area, then this raises questions about how it is to be judged. What does research tell us about how partnership working might have contributed to the dynamics of the NHS?

Dickinson and Glasby (2010, in particular page 819) provide an excellent summary of common themes in the research on partnerships around six main issues:

- the failure to identify desired outcomes (so partnership become an end rather than a means to an end);
- calling the new entity a 'partnership' when it is really a 'takeover';
- claiming that the partnership was meant to provide better services when it was really about organisational self-interest;
- seeking to achieve unstated aspirations while articulating a different set of aspirations publicly;
- the tendency to see partnership working as a panacea to current problems and placing too much faith in partnerships to deliver over-ambitious aspirations, risking disillusionment, and;
- undermining the partnership by not attending to practical details.

The authors stress that 'the same sorts of problems and issues tend to crop up time and time again within local health and social care communities that are attempting to establish partnerships' (2010, p 826). Glasby et al (2011) point to the importance of joint working between health and social care especially, and again emphasise the need for partnerships to be outcomes-focused, concerned with the depth and breadth of their relationships, and of the need to work together on different levels. They point to structural, procedural, financial and professional barriers, and the importance of shared vision, clarity of roles and responsibilities, and the need for accountability for joint working (2011, p 6). Indeed, if we compare the issues that they raise with those listed by Hudson and Hardy (2002) nearly 10 years earlier, there is remarkable commonality.

Hunter and Perkins (2012), examining partnership working in public health, find many of the same barriers in place, and that less formal and more organic partnerships tend to be more successful, but also raise the key finding that the continual policy and organisational 'churn' in place in the NHS was making it difficult to establish and sustain the long-term relationships on which partnerships were dependent. This finding is also a central part of the message from a reflective piece from Hudson (2012, p 123), who, looking back over 20 years of his own research, concludes that 'Although localities have on occasion commendably attempted to develop joint strategies and integrated provision, they have always been doing so in an unhelpful political and policy environment which has failed to fundamentally challenge silo working, failed to understand the nature of effective partnering and has yet harboured unrealistic expectations of what could be achieved.' It is hard to think of a more effective summary.

Assessing the programme theory of choice and competition

The empirical work on patient choice suggests that it is facing considerable problems in implementation, and the econometric research, while pointing to important changes in clinical outcomes and patient referral outcomes since 2006, is unable to attribute those results to either choice or competition.

In terms of our programme theory, there seems to be evidence that patient choice has only had a 'limited' impact on the NHS so far (Dixon and Robertson, 2011, p 63), with many organisations not reporting choice as being important in their decision-making that was based more on targets and NSFs (Dixon and Jones, 2011, p 134).

There is some evidence, however, of rural patients more used to travel being prepared to make greater use of choice (even if this might lead to potential inequalities), but in general 'patients are extremely loyal to local providers' (Dixon and Robertson, 2011, p 64). Competition appears to have had some effect, but 'it did not improve productivity enough to offset the resource increases' and 'the NHS budget was growing rapidly, taking the edge off competitive pressures' (Mays and Dixon, 2011, p 133). Indeed, it is surely time to ask whether the costs of NHS reorganisations putting competition as their basis since 1989 have achieved anything like the health improvements that could have resulted from simply spending that money on more care. The effect of PbR is hard to disentangle from that of competition and choice (as they are hard, in turn, to disentangle from one another), but again, the costs of introduction and administration of the system have been substantial and not fully documented (Farrar et al, 2011), giving us reason to wonder whether they exceed any benefits that might be attributable to its use.

If the programme theory for choice and competition was meant to lead to patients and GPs making informed choices about care referrals, it is hard to see how this is even possible given the time constraints in appointment times, and that neither patients nor GPs seem to make much use of information systems when making referrals. Referral patterns have not changed dramatically, and outside of rural areas, most patients have not been prepared to travel further for their care. If patients were meant to be driving choice and competition, then evidence from GP surgeries suggests that they are not being widely consulted about their referral preferences. It is extremely difficult to reconcile econometric research, suggesting that providers performing well are receiving more care referrals with empirical research of the choice process itself, but there are substantial reasons to doubt that choice and competition are driving care improvements in themselves.

In sum, it is hard to see that the programme theory for choice and competition has worked very well in the 2000s, with choice not being widely taken up by patients (who do not use the information systems that are meant to be underpinning the process), competition not leading to many tangible results, and the transaction costs of the system being substantial.

Comparing the internal market of the 1990s with the mixed economy of care in the 2000s

The 1990s programme theory for patient choice and competition was that, by positioning providers (hospitals) and purchasers (district health authorities and GP fundholders) in a dynamic relationship with one another, the latter would drive up the quality of care through more careful purchasing, and the former would compete with one another to earn contracts.

However, what seems to have happened was that there was little 'market-making' from purchasers, who continued to behave much as before in terms of their contracting, and little competition between providers, as there were few real competitors in each local healthcare system, and patients were generally reluctant to travel far for their care.

The model of choice and competition in the 2000s was different in that it attempted to increase competition through the entry of non-public providers, purchasing was to be done on a fixed-price basis to try and put an increased emphasis on raising quality, and there was to be a more flexible payments system to avoid the block contracts of the 1990s. Equally, rather more emphasis was put on patient choice, and the provision of more information to allow informed choices to be made (through patient choice leaflets and the NHS Choices website). The programme theory for the 2000s was that by giving patients and GPs more information and greater opportunity to make choices, along with a payment system designed to link resources to those choices (on the demand side), and by introducing greater competition between providers through the entry of non-public providers and a system of fixing prices so that care could be compared in terms of quality (on the supply side), a more responsive, efficient and effective means of organising and paying for care could be achieved.

However, what seems to have happened is that there has not been widespread non-public entry into the new market for care (so limiting competition), that patients have remained (except in a few settings) reluctant to travel far or change their healthcare provider (either GP or hospital), or to make use of information systems supporting care referral choices. Perhaps more importantly from a market-based logic, public providers in particular have not been allowed to 'fail' (so removing the incentive to compete more strongly), perhaps in recognition that they effectively underpin NHS care provision in terms of both scale and scope.

The comparison of the 1990s and 2000s is summarised below, in Table 5.2.

Table 5.2: Patient choice and competition in the 1990s and 2000s

	1990s	2000s
Competition between	Public providers	Public providers and new non-public entrants
Basis of competition	Price and quality (limited)	Fixed price and quality (limited)
Contract type	Block	Some block, move to lower scales (money follows the patient through PbR)
Purchasers	District health authorities GP fundholders	PCTs Practice-based commissioners
Incentives for gaining contracts	Limited – no real resource pressure	Some – increased focus on budgets, but financial failure rare
Incentives for awarding contracts well	Limited – not much competition, sticky contractual arrangements GP fundholders – keep some of surplus	Slightly wider – some entry but basis of market predominantly local with limited competition No real incentive for generating surplus
Quality of information	Poor	A little better – but not really used by patients or GPs
Role of choice	Referral to secondary care (especially hospital)	Referral to secondary care Attempt to expand to GP choice Attempt to expand to public health

The mixed economy of care of the 2000s attempted to learn the lessons of the internal market of the 1990s, and did address many of the failings of the previous decade. But we still can't compare the costs of introducing the system with the limited benefits it has achieved, and were we able to do so, it seems extremely unlikely that it could be judged a success. Had we simply spent the billions involved in setting up and implementing PbR, Choose and Book and NHS Choices on extra care instead, it seems likely this would have created a substantial net gain.

If choice and competition have not been a success, what about the second part of the local dynamic programme theory – increasing PPI?

Patient and public involvement and participation in the NHS

The second mechanism by which local dynamic reorganisation was attempted in the NHS in England during the 2000s was through a series of changes to the institutions and organisations of PPI. These changes are meant to be complementary to the choice and competition-based reorganisations explored above, in that they are based on 'voice'-type mechanisms (Hirschmann, 1970).

Incorporating patient and public voice into healthcare is a local dynamic programme theory that suggests that in order for health services to generate self-sustaining improvements they must better incorporate the views of those they are meant to serve. Therefore, a range of mechanisms needs to be put in place to capture not only individual patient views of the service they have received, but also to involve the public more generally in the governance of health services. By being more responsive to individual patient needs (in a more consumerist role, in many respects), and to the wishes of local publics (in a more citizen-type role, by members of the public serving as representatives of their communities), health services can be improved to become more responsive to patient wishes and more democratic, in line with public preferences.

Improving PPI in the NHS was a recurring theme for the Labour government from 1999 onwards (Davies et al, 1999). This approach was elaborated in the NHS Plan a year later (Secretary of State for Health, 2000), and again in *Shifting the balance of power* (DH, 2001d), which aimed to give local communities greater influence over the development of services, especially through engagement with the newly introduced PCTs.

The institutional structures through which greater PPI was to be achieved underwent considerable change between 1997 and 2010. When Labour came to power, involvement and participation of patients and the public occurred mainly through the community health councils set up in the 1974 reforms. These organisations used a diverse range of means to attempt to influence and improve local healthcare, often achieving adverse local publicity when health service organisations were seen to be failing their patients, or helping organise campaigns against poor practice (Klein, 2006). However, there were few statutory duties for health services to consult with their local communities or patients, and the government sought a more pro-active approach to involving the public.

Labour's 2001 Health and Social Care Act put in place a requirement for NHS organisations to involve and consult with the public in the planning of services and the development of proposals for changes in the way those services were provided. Equally, as noted in the discussion on central control reorganisation, foundation trusts were made accountable to their local community by having membership schemes in which the public could participate in their governance.

The NHS and Health Care Professions Act 2002 abolished community health councils (a move regarded as being controversial at the time, with some prominent community health councils lobbying hard against their closure), replacing them with PPIFs, one for each PCT in England, and managed by the CPPIH. Local PPIFs also worked with local government overview and scrutiny committees to attempt to hold local health services in each area to account (Hughes et al, 2009). In 2003, the Health and Social Care (Community Health and Standards) Act set up the Healthcare Commission (which took over the duties of the CHI, which had subsequently become the Commission for Healthcare Audit and Inspection in the meantime), and whose responsibilities included conducting patient surveys and involving patient groups in local service user consultation. Finally, the Local Government and Public Involvement in Health Act 2007 abolished PPIFs and replaced them with LINks, which were established in April 2008, before being abolished in the coalition government's 2010 reorganisation.

As in many other areas, the Labour government's approach to reorganisation in the area of PPI appeared rather hyperactive, and gives us real difficulties in evaluating whether all these changes were successful or not – it is hard to measure something that is continually being reorganised. However, we can assess what research has to say about the extent to PPI organisations (in all their forms) achieved the outcomes specified in the programme theory above.

What does the research on patient and public involvement tell us?

A first research finding suggests that the abolition of community health councils, which had been in place for over 25 years, resulted in a loss of expertise in public participation (Barnes et al, 2003), with staff not being allowed to transfer from the old representative organisations to the new ones, such as PALS (Baggott, 2005; Dent and Haslam, 2006). The new institutions established appeared to have few clear guidelines as to how they were meant to be functioning, and lacked the resources to do the jobs that were asked of them (Forster and Gabe, 2008). If the reorganisation was meant to standardise public involvement and to raise the standards of areas with poorly functioning community health councils, the result was a plurality of very different models of participation from one locality to the next. In some areas they were based on bureaucratic models that favoured expert opinion rather than public consultation, while others were more participative and dialogic, allowing wider and deeper consultation to take place (Callaghan and Wistow, 2006a, 2006b).

The participatory mechanisms introduced in the early 2000s have also been criticised on the grounds that their goals were confused. They were, their critics claimed, not designed to make health services more democratic (Barnes et al, 2003), but instead were based on a more limited, smaller-scale view of service improvement, and so lacked independence and legitimacy as a result (Forster and Gabe, 2008). The 2008 Monitor report to the House of Commons Health Select Committee suggested that there was a lack of evidence that foundation trusts had promoted either greater innovation or increased PPI.

A general criticism of the government's entire approach to PPI during the decade was that it did not take sufficient account of the different motivations of different public groups to be involved in their local health services (Barnes et al, 2003). Equally, there seemed to be conceptual confusion from the government in their use of consumerist language to justify patient choice reforms, but at the same time attempts to position the public as citizens through their reforms of participatory mechanisms (Forster and Gabe, 2008). Consumerist and citizen-type involvement can be complementary when based on a consumer-model of improvement, and the focus is on service responsiveness to individual need. This can be the case because, if services are responsive to all individuals, they will also be responsive to patients as a whole. However, where individual patients are able to make services more responsive to their needs at the expense of other patients, then consumer-type involvement runs the risk of favouring patients who are able to show 'sharp elbows' rather than working for everyone.

Public participation mechanisms are based on a different kind of mechanism to individual consumer-based models, with members of the public attempting to act in more collectivist, representational, citizen-type roles to try and improve services. Where governments conflate consumer representation and public participation, this has the potential to cause confusion, and is illustrated in mental health where service users resisted being labelled as consumers through the use of self-organising groups that campaigned to be heard through voice-type mechanisms for service improvement instead (Bolzan et al, 2001; Bolzan and Gale, 2002). In his study of public involvement in cancer genetics services, Martin (2008b) found that while clinical staff were prepared to listen to members of the public in participatory meetings, public members found their roles restrictive, with professionals positioning them as consumers of services. At the same time, the professionals expected the public to be deferential to their professional status. The public, on the other hand, wanted to be equal participants in the decision-making processes, and to become stakeholders in the way that services developed in the future. A key finding from research into consumer roles in other public services (Clarke, 2005; Clarke et al, 2007) suggests that members of the public who want to take on broader, 'voice' roles often find themselves frustrated as they are limited by the way they are regarded as individual 'consumers' instead.

A first issue in this area, then, is that it is often mired in confusion over exactly what governments mean by 'participation' or 'involvement', with consumer and citizen-type roles being conflated.

Expectations of involvement

Research on patient involvement from the UK as well as from other countries suggests that the public, health service management and clinicians often have very different expectations about the extent of public involvement that can be achieved through participatory mechanisms. This finding is perhaps clearest in a Canadian study from Abelson and colleagues (Abelson et al, 2004), but is confirmed by UK-based research on participation. Abelson's work is summarised in a table from their work, in Table 5.3 below.

Abelson's work suggests that the public, when asked to participate in health services, need to understand the wider context of the decision they are being asked to be involved in. They also need to understand the link between the consultation that is taking place, and the outcome of the decision that is being made, not least because they do not wish to be involved in processes that are simply 'talking shop', with little actual influence over the final decision (Stoker, 2006). The public expect a careful recruitment process to try and achieve an appropriate mix of people, and then to be involved in power sharing with decision-makers and an open process that encourages impartiality rather than the imposition of rule-based discussion. Finally, they expect full, open, information sharing to establish trust, with that information being presented to them through neutral facilitators, time to build confidence with the topic under consideration, and a combination of lay and expert views rather than listening only to what decision-makers regard as 'credible and trusted sources'. The list of requirements and expectations in the column on the right in Table 5.3, which identifies what citizens want from consultation and participation processes, is both more extensive and more demanding than those that inform the design principles presented in the column on the left, which reflects

Table 5.3: Comparison of public consultation design principles with citizens' views about public involvement

Public consultation design principles	Citizens' views about public involvement
Clearly communicate	*Communication*
The purpose of the consultation	Clear communication about the purpose of the consultation and its relationship to the larger decision-making process
Its procedural rules	Identifiable links between the consultation and the decision outcome
Represent views, interests and constituencies	*People*
By carefully considering whose input should be considered	Careful recruitment of the appropriate mix of people for the issue being discussed
Develop procedural rules	*Process*
That promote power sharing and mutual respect among participants That allow for adequate in questions, clarification, listening and understanding That promote trust, credibility and legitimacy	Promote power sharing and mutual respect among participants and between participants and decision-makers through neutral, impartial facilitation
Provide information	*Information exchange*
That is accessible Presented in a way that informs discussion That can be discussed and interpreted From credible and trusted sources	Information sharing in a context of trust Information to be presented clearly, honestly and with integrity Needs to ensure participants' comfort with the topic and to build confidence for meaningful participation Lay views and experiential expertise should be listened to and considered

Source: Abelson et al (2004, p 211)

what they are most likely to experience in such exercises in public organisations.

On the ground, UK-based research on the use of approaches to public involvement such as that of citizens' juries has shown the difficulties of getting participatory decision-making to work (Pickard, 1998). More importantly, and in line with the findings from Abelson, where members of the public are asked to be involved in a decision in which they regard they have no say, or they can see no link between the participatory method and the actual decision, they find the process disempowering, and this can serve to deter them from getting involved again (Pickard, 1998).

There are case studies of strong practice in public participation that can be used both to demonstrate how it can be done better by the

NHS, as well as simply showing that deep and longer-term engagement of citizens in their local health services is possible (Wistow, 2001; Callaghan and Wistow, 2006a, 2006b). It does appear, however, that such examples appear relatively infrequently in the research, and so remain the exception rather than the rule.

An area where health services seek public involvement, but which has a strong overlap with a consumer-type role, is that of patient complaints. These are important because they have the potential to bridge both citizen and consumer roles, depending on whether such feedback is treated as a source of potential service improvement for the organisation against which they are directed, or no attempt to aggregate complaints is made, so that learning lost. Sadly, it seems that NHS organisations are often still struggling to deal with complaints, even at the individual patient level. There are concerns that NHS trusts of all types are becoming more secretive in dealing with complaints, and that the processes involved in complaining are still lengthy, onerous and time-consuming for patients to engage with, with little opportunity to challenge trusts where they find against the complaint, or for personal interactions between patients and health professionals to achieve resolutions outside of complaints processes (Allsop and Jones, 2008). In any case, poor treatment of complaints appears to represent a huge missed opportunity for using patient voice to improve health services. At Mid Staffordshire, the failure to deal with complaints and patient voice was a central part of the story presented in the Francis Report (Francis, 2013).

Representation and democracy

PPI processes also raise questions about representation and democracy for health services. In terms of representation, and as noted above, Abelson suggests that the public place a strong emphasis on the need for an appropriate mix of people to put together, but formal, governmental processes often attempt to achieve groups that are representative of local communities in some form. Martin (2008a, 2008b, 2009) and Learmonth et al (2009) point out how difficult it has been for members to be representative of diverse communities (and 'community' has itself been ill defined in government policies), to have a democratic role, and also be an expert with many professional traits such as having sufficient time to devote to the organisation and specialist expertise. These difficulties lead to tensions — the choice of which members of the public are chosen in participative forums is central to their legitimacy (Barnes et al, 2003) — but it is often not clear exactly how that legitimacy is being established through representation (Forster and Gabe, 2008; Learmonth et al, 2009), and members of the public often seek to distance themselves from being in any way representative of a wider group, wanting to stress their own experiences and background instead (Mitton et al, 2009).

In terms of democracy, and of the link between NHS organisations and local authorities, local authority overview and scrutiny committees were meant to help bridge the gap and make health services more accountable, but this was an indirect democratic link only, without direct electoral relationships between the NHS and local authorities. There was enthusiasm in local government for using scrutiny committees as a means of achieving greater local involvement in health services (and local government more generally), but they struggled to establish the rules, support and local relationships that might have made them effective (Hamer, 2003). It was also less than clear how different participation committees were meant to draw boundaries of responsibility and accountability (Forster and Gabe, 2008) with the abolition of PPIFs due to criticism about their inability to represent local communities. Their replacements, LINks, appear to have further confused the means by which services were meant to be held democratically accountable (Dixon et al, 2010a). Research suggests that PALS were too small and too detached from clinical governance to cause meaningful change, and their lack of democratic accountability meant they could be seen 'as a means of manipulating patients and the public rather than empowering them' (Baggott, 2005, p 546).

Lessons from public and patient involvement programmes in the 2000s

A first observation about attempts to achieve public and patient participation during the 2000s is that it was an area of almost continuous reorganisation, with little opportunity for the new organisations put in place by the government (be they PPIFs or LINks) to become established and embedded in the governance structures of local health areas so they were able to represent the public's interest in some sense.

That there were three different organisational forms in a decade (which began with community health councils) meant that continuity was difficult to establish and learning lost as participatory mechanisms were undergoing reorganisation. Each change has taken time, to recruit new members and embed new organisations in relation to other health and social public sector bodies such as local authorities and NHS trusts.

The introduction of LINks in particular resulted in 'something of a vacuum' due to the slow process of change (Coleman et al, 2009, p 25).

An important finding is that the public want deeper and more meaningful participation than the NHS is generally able to offer. Research suggests that the public want to be more equal partners in decision-making processes than token representatives of their communities who are only consulted about decisions they believe have already been made. The link between consultation and the final decision needs to be made clear to members of the public so that they believe their time and participation is valued. Although it is clearly not the case that the public can be consulted on all aspects of decision-making in large, complex healthcare organisations, where they are asked to participate they need to be given the time and resources to do so. This finding links to work examining the role of the public in democratic processes more generally that suggests it is crucial that expectations are clearly set up, and the public are given the space and time to make meaningful contributions (Stoker, 2006). Members of the public want to be selected based on their individual traits rather than as representatives of communities, and to be able to make meaningful contributions when they do give their time.

At present, it seems that the NHS is not good at treating patient feedback or complaints as a 'voice' mechanism for service improvement, and the reorganisations of the 2000s have created confusion as to how the consumer and citizen roles expected of patients are meant to be combined. It seems that the NHS is still struggling to put in place organisations or routes by which the public can improve health services through being involved in decision-making.

By 2010, a further reorganisation of participation mechanisms was occurring, this time proposing new organisations called Healthwatch that would replace LINks. This was regarded not as a means of achieving greater public involvement or representation, but instead as consumer representative bodies, and so had different goals to either PPIFs or LINks. Healthwatch is placing an emphasis on the consumer rather than citizen role (DH, 2013), and moving further away from the deeper participative models that the research above suggests the public are seeking.

Revisiting the programme theory for patient and public involvement

If PPI is about improving health services by better incorporating the views of those the services are meant to be serving, the reorganisations of the 2000s do not appear to have been a success. Again, Mid Staffordshire shows NHS organisations at their worst in being able to ignore patient concerns and complaints. Patient voices were not being taken seriously, and public involvement in services was not being used as a means of challenging and improving practice. Such failings were compounded by a LINks organisation that was dysfunctional and achieved no constructive work at all (Francis, 2013, Exec summary).

The Francis Inquiry into Mid Staffordshire (2013) recommends improved training for Healthwatch members, national consistency in structures and sufficient funds released from local authorities to provide independence, but initial signs are not encouraging. Local authorities have, in some instances, curtailed funding for the new organisations, and new host organisations have been appointed for some local Healthwatch organisations through competitive tendering. Far from this being the smooth evolution from LINks that was outlined in policy documents, the reality for some areas has been yet another hiatus (or vacuum) of several months while new organisations get up and running. LINks have produced 'legacy documents' in an attempt to preserve what has been learned. However, it remains to be seen how far these are actually used and how much organisational memory is lost.

In order for the programme theory of PPI to work, members of the public have to be given a genuine opportunity to participate at the level they wish – which appears to be at a more extensive and engaged level than the one that health services too often presently give them – and that they are able to move beyond consumer-type roles to be able to work with health services across a broader range of issues than such roles allow. But the NHS does not have a good record of treating individual patient voices seriously – in dealing with complaints efficiently and learning from them, or in engaging the public in the running of health services at the depth they want. There are examples of good practice in each area that can be learned from, but they seem few and far between.

Comparing local dynamic mechanisms in the 2000s

Attempts at local dynamic reorganisation in healthcare aim to put in place mechanisms by which improvements can be self-sustaining, in contrast to top-down reorganisations that require a central agency or organisation to exert control. The extension of patient choice and the reinstatement of the market mechanism in healthcare, and the almost continuous changes to PPI, were the main attempts by the government to achieve local dynamic reorganisation.

The government's approach to patient choice and competition highlights confusion as to whether it is genuinely patients who are meant to be driving improvements in care through their choices, or whether GPs are meant to be doing this on their behalf. PbR, with its linking of referral care decisions with payment, was meant to put in place an incentive for good providers to compete in or enter new health economies, as there was the potential for resources to follow care choices, but this only worked if good providers could be identified, and if GPs and patients chose them, and there appear to be considerable barriers to both of these things happening. Perhaps even more significantly, in a time of resource frugality in the 2010s, rather than the growth of the 2000s, it implies that poor providers of care, or those that are unable to attract sufficient care contracts, should be allowed to become bankrupt, and even close – in the words of Dixon and Mays (2011, p 160), 'policy-makers need to decide whether the extension and development of the market is suited to a period of consolidation and dramatic financial tightening'. It would be ironic if market-type mechanisms don't work at allocating scarce resources, as that is meant to be their role in the economy in general.

Choice and competition model therefore raises difficult issues, not only about how informed choices about care referrals can be made and operationalised when GPs appear unwilling or unable to refer to providers based on the best quality information, but also where patients appear reluctant to travel to attend referral appointments, whether policy-makers are prepared to face the consequences of public providers potentially facing financial failure, and closure when there is a definite political cost to such decisions.

That choice and competition requiring informed care referrals is a problem because, at present, neither GPs nor patients appear to routinely make use of care outcomes data in order to decide which care provider should be chosen. GPs simply do not have the time to be experts on every possible provider they can refer patients to, and service-level data is not as accessible or available as it needs to be. Patients, on the other hand, have an extra problem in that they are often asked to make referral decisions with little or no information at all, with very little support, and in contexts such as time-limited GP appointments or on the telephone that are hardly conducive to good decision-making. Given these problems, a competitive marketplace for care does not seem structured to lead to informed choices being made, and so it is hardly surprising that, even where major clinical failings are happening, GPs continue to refer patients to those providers, and patients do not seem to object. Indeed, even after the care failings at

Mid Staffordshire, there were public protests in April 2013 about even a planned scaling back of services there.

The second question, whether policy-makers are prepared to face the consequences of PbR leading to public-provider financial failure, has yet to be fully tested, but the coalition government has already bailed out public hospital trusts facing deficits due to PFI contracts to the tune of £1.5 billion, and so the signs are that they will not allow the care market to work to its final logic. This is not surprising – politicians have faced considerable electoral consequences for threatening to close local hospitals, losing by-elections to single-issue campaigners, and so will have to ask themselves difficult questions before allowing a closure to occur. Equally, without a significant local public provider, the care market may lack sufficient capacity to fully meet local demand as well as lacking a provider of last resort should non-public providers elect to leave the market. As such, there are both political and pragmatic reasons why public providers may not be allowed to financially fail, and if such exit is not possible, then this works directly against the imposition of the market logic.

At the patient level, it still seems there is a preference for the guarantee of good local services rather than a wish to choose healthcare providers, and that when patients want a greater say over their care, it is often because they have a long-term condition that allows them to become expert patients in their own right. Equally, patients may well want the kind of choice they are not being offered – a choice of when they will be seen rather than which provider will see them.

Confusion over exactly who is meant to be making choices to drive the healthcare market are increased by the 2010/12 reorganisation, which puts at its heart GP-led commissioning groups purchasing care – suggesting that, at a minimum, GPs will decide who they purchase care from, and then patients will be able to make choices within those contracts. But whether GPs have the capacity to negotiate such contracts without making extensive use of commissioning support organisations – moving care referral decisions away from GPs when the legitimacy of the reforms appears to be based on moving such decisions as close to patients as possible – is open to question. Indeed, by 2015 commissioning support organisations can be outsourced entirely to the private sector, raising difficult issues about how they will remain accountable. Equally, how patients are meant to make decisions about to whom they would like their care to be referred without good information, support and time, is again, not clear, especially given that they may not want to make such choices in the first place. We return to this topic when considering the prospects for the coalition government's NHS reorganisation in Chapters Six and Seven.

Patient and public participation mechanisms have been under a process of almost continual reorganisation since 2001, but appear to be equally mired in conceptual confusion. Rather than allowing deep participation where the public are treated as joint decision-makers and where the link between participation and the final decision is made clear, participatory mechanisms are often based on consultation or tokenistic representation, missing the opportunity to gain a more full public perspective on governance issues. Attempts to achieve greater public involvement by making them members of foundation trusts appear to have resulted in little improvement in these terms. By 2008, commentators regarded participatory mechanisms in healthcare as being in disarray (Bradshaw, 2008), and since then, yet another round of reorganisation has been proposed.

In both choice and participatory mechanisms the model proposed in reorganisation appears to be increasingly consumerist, based on a model in which dialogic or collectivist answers to improving care are rejected, and individualistic, transactional models are favoured instead. In patient choice, decisions often have to be made on the basis of little information in a short space of time, with patient choice advisers not being rolled out in the national policy implementation despite the Office of Public Sector Reform making clear this was necessary (2005). What both GPs and patients appear to want are consultations based on mutual respect and dialogue rather than the transactional model of choice which appears to be emerging (McCartney, 2012). In participatory mechanisms, the deeper participation models that the public suggest they want are being moved increasingly onto an individualistic, consumer-based model.

As such, neither of the local dynamic mechanisms designed to achieve service improvement appear to be based on what patients or doctors want, and are limited in their ability to achieve the greater responsiveness of health services successive governments have aimed for. Considering that such proposals lie at the heart of the coalition government's healthcare reorganisation, there must be significant concerns about their prospects for achieving their goal of improving health services in England.

SIX

The prospects for NHS reorganisation post-2010

Introduction

> But of all the changes that were enacted by the 2012 Health and Social Care Act, the decision to abolish a large proportion of the organisations that comprise the NHS in order to replace them with a whole new set of organisations that only those with the most arcane interest in NHS management structures will ever be able to tell apart is probably the least useful. (Taylor, 2013, pp 85-6)

Chapter One opened with a quote from Roger Taylor suggesting that NHS reorganisations have achieved little other than changes in 'letterheads and job titles'. What the evidence presented in the first five chapters suggests is that the common currency of healthcare reorganisation contains rather fewer examples of successful change than we might hope. There are, however, also some successes from which we can learn.

This book has considered research examining the NHS reorganisations of the 1980s and 1990s, and in more depth, those attempted by Labour, especially during the 2000s, elaborating the central control and local dynamic programme theories that underpinned their reorganisations of the NHS in England during that decade, to produce more detailed accounts of what appears to work, and also how, and under what circumstances.

Although central control mechanisms have been shown to be problematic in hospital settings, the QOF in the area of general practice has shown there is potential for their adaptation. Local dynamic mechanisms, such as patient choice and competition, and PPI, demonstrate isolated examples of working well, but are areas where it is far more difficult to produce a detailed programme theory that shows how reorganisation can work well because of the significant problems they have encountered in both policy design and implementation.

This chapter explores what these elaborated programme theories can tell us about NHS reform after 2010. Following the general election that year, the coalition government put in place a radical programme of reorganisation for the NHS in England, courting significant controversy in the process, and resulting in changes that have been referred to as the most significant in the history of the NHS (Hunter, 2011). This chapter considers the nature of the coalition government's reorganisation, and the prospects for it working based on research evidence from previous chapters.

The NHS in the last years of the Labour government

By 2010 the Labour government had been in power for 13 years, and much of the momentum for the reform of its domestic policy appeared to have been lost (Rawnsley, 2010). In June 2007 Tony Blair stepped aside as Prime Minister, and Gordon Brown took over as both leader of the Labour Party and Prime Minister. Brown's timing was to prove dreadful. After a brief honeymoon period that appeared to show a change in direction, moving away from concern with policy presentation that had been so central to the New Labour project (including the memorable phrase 'not flash, just Gordon'), Brown found himself having to deal with the worst economic crisis since the 1930s, and at the centre of world-level discussions about how the financial system might be supported. Domestic reform moved away from being the government's central priority (Richards, 2010).

From 2007 to 2010, there was a distinctive final movement in Labour's health reform agenda. If the period 1997-2000 was one in which Labour attempted to make conciliatory gestures to the medical profession after the antagonism with the Conservative government during the early 1990s, 2000-02 was one in which performance management and top-down reform predominated, and 2003-07 saw the reintroduction of the mixed economy of care, then 2007-10 seems to have seen a return to advocating a more pragmatic approach to the healthcare market.

After 2007, Secretary of State, Andy Burnham, much to the frustration of pro-market advocates such as Norman Warner (2011), appeared unenthusiastic about greater non-public provision in the NHS and wanted to give public providers a 'preferred' status in the marketplace that suggested that the effects of the market for care would be somewhat constrained. Although market mechanisms were certainly not rolled back, they did not appear to be as enthusiastically implemented or progressed as they had been up to 2007, with little growth in non-public provision and little sense from detailed fieldwork in public organisations that markets were at the forefront of managers' minds (Dixon et al, 2010b, p 134).

At the 2010 election, Labour's election manifesto suggested that, if they were re-elected, there would be an extension of the use of individual budgets in healthcare, but there was no sign of further significant NHS reorganisation. Individual budgets had been piloted in social care, and involved giving patients a set sum of cash each year to buy their own treatment, independent of local authority control (Baxter et al, 2011), and there appeared to be an all-party consensus about extending non-public provision in healthcare (Timmins, 2012). Instead of stressing greater competition in the NHS, Labour also promised to put in place measures to get better coordination and integration between health and social care services. The Conservatives published a manifesto that – despite suggestions in opposition from Shadow Secretary of State for Health, Andrew Lansley, that he had more radical plans – offered little that was really new, but had as its centrepiece a promise to maintain NHS expenditure levels that Labour felt unable to match. This put the Brown government on the back foot in election discussions over the NHS – an unusual position for the Labour Party to find itself in, given its status as the political party that 'created' the NHS.

During the 2010 election campaign, the NHS was hardly mentioned – Labour appeared nervous of raising it because of the Conservative promise to maintain funding for the NHS, and the Conservatives did not seem to want to press home their advantage in that area or discuss their plans for the NHS in more detail (Timmins, 2012). Andrew Lansley barely featured in the Conservative campaign, and the NHS was not a central issue. The public were more concerned with the nation's economic woes.

The 2010 coalition government

After the 2010 election result there was a brief hiatus while the major political parties, for the first time in a generation, attempted to form a coalition government. The eventual result, in which the largest party by seats, the Conservatives, joined with the smallest major political party, the Liberal Democrats, to form a new government, then published its coalition agreement (HM Government, 2010). In this they sought to combine a range of Conservative ideas including the creation of an independent NHS board in an apparent attempt to remove health from direct political interference by allocating resources and providing commissioning guidelines independent of government, and turning

Monitor, its foundation trust regulator, into an economic regulator to take charge of and oversee the market management function, including access, competition and price-setting in the NHS (Timmins, 2012). The document promised to 'stop the top-down reorganisations of the NHS that have got in the way of patient care', but suggested that PCTs should include a stronger element of local democracy (probably as a concession to the Liberal Democrats). The proposals, put together by the influential Conservative Oliver Letwin and Liberal Democrat Danny Alexander, appeared to suggest that the NHS was not going to be a central focus of governmental activity, and that any change was likely to be less radical than the government's proposals in terms of social security reform in reducing benefits, and education reform in relation to its 'free schools' agenda.

However, barely six weeks later, the new coalition government published its *Liberating the NHS* White Paper (Secretary of State for Health, 2010) that proposed a far more radical reorganisation. Lansley, apparently believing the proposals in the coalition agreement could not possibly work as they mixed local democracy with market mechanisms and an independent board, proposed a very different approach.

Lansley's plans abolished PCTs and strategic health authorities, with GPs taking over all commissioning (with a reduced role for NICE in overseeing their decisions), an autonomous commissioning board coordinating purchasing decisions where necessary, and a new economic regulator put in place to promote competition. Patients were to be given a choice of 'any willing provider' for their care, management costs were to be cut, public health transferred to local government, and health and wellbeing boards set up to try and join up GP commissioning with that of social care and public health.

The model proposed by Lansley had a theoretical elegance in that it took Labour's pre-2007 model for the mixed economy of care and attempted to move it onto its next logical stage, insisting that competition between public and non-public providers was the best way of improving care, and that the market needed to be insulated from government interference in order to work. As such, it was based very much on extension of the choice and competition programme theory that had been in place under Labour.

Missing from the White Paper, however, was a narrative explaining why the reorganisation was necessary at a time when public approval ratings for the NHS were at an all-time high, or how, combined with the reorganisation, the NHS was going to find the £20 billion of efficiency savings by 2014 which the new government required of it (Timmins, 2012).

After a period during which the medical profession appeared at least unsure, and sometimes even cautiously welcoming of the White Paper, opposition to the reorganisation steadily grew. Support continued to come from bodies such as the National Association for Primary Care that saw the reorganisation as holding the potential to increase their ability to purchase good care for their patients. Opposition grew as medical and nursing representative bodies appeared to realise the size of the changes, and were unable to understand why a reorganisation of the scale required was necessary or even viable. This opposition was arguably led by the Royal College of General Practitioners after Clare Gerada became its chair. Gerada argued that the reorganisation represented nothing less than the privatisation of the NHS.

Even within the coalition government, senior Liberal Democrats such as Baroness Shirley Williams expressed concerns about the proposals, and applied considerable pressure on her party leader Nick Clegg to re-examine them. The House of Commons Health Select Committee, under the chairmanship of a Conservative member and former Secretary of State for Health, Stephen Dorrell, made it clear that they were not convinced by the government's plans.

Opponents of the reorganisation raised a range of concerns in addition to the allegations that it amounted to privatising the NHS. In particular there were concerns about the lack of clarity around how GPs would acquire the expertise to commission care, the move to make the NHS more independent of government and how parliamentary and democratic accountability would be ensured under such a system. By March 2011 the British Medical Association was proposing, in a special representative meeting, that the bill be dropped, and 38 Degrees, a web-based membership campaigning organisation, used Twitter and Facebook to publicise a campaign to get over 100,000 electronic signatures on a petition to get a House of Commons debate on the bill (ironically a process put in place by the coalition government itself to try and achieve more public engagement with politics).

At the beginning of April 2011, just as the bill completed its committee stage in Parliament, the government announced a 'pause' to 'listen, engage and amend' its content. The NHS Future Forum was appointed to those ends, and was headed by Steve Field, Clare Gerada's predecessor at the Royal College of General Practitioners. The Future Forum's report (2011) led to the government proposing over 1,000 amendments to the bill.

Under the oversight of the then NHS Chief Executive, David Nicholson, a much more bureaucratic structure was put in place in which local commissioning bodies would oversee GP commissioning.

In many respects they looked remarkably like a stripped-down reinvention of the abolished PCTs. In the House of Lords arguments about competition and accountability led to a total of over 2,000 amendments being passed even as an increasing range of medical representative bodies came out in opposition to the bill. There was even an argument from Conservative supporters that the bill should be dropped as it was turning into the government's 'poll tax' and so likely to lose them the next election (Montgomerie, 2012), and there was also the strange sight of former Labour Secretary of State Alan Milburn suggesting that the 'debacle' of the NHS reorganisation was in danger of losing the market-based gains achieved by the previous government (Milburn, 2011).

After its difficult passage through both Houses, the Health and Social Care Act came on to the statute book in March 2012. The government, however, had expended a huge amount of time, effort and political capital in its NHS reorganisation, and in the face of widespread public bemusement at what was going on, or why an NHS reorganisation was necessary, with only 20 per cent of the public rating the NHS as the most important issue facing Britain in February 2012 in an *Economist* and Ipsos MORI poll.

Where does this leave us?

The final form of the Health and Social Care Act, after 2,000 amendments and all the political furore, appears to be a compromise between Lansley's original vision of a market-led NHS, and its opponents' amendments reflecting concerns about the reorganisation proceeding too quickly, a lack of political accountability in the new structures and excessive competition.

First, clinical commissioning groups (CCGs) (through which GPs will commission care) will be GP-led rather than GP-run, and have statutory duties to engage with a wide range of health organisations and interest groups about their plans. This is some distance from an entrepreneurial model of care purchasing, and within the context of the multilayered commissioning structure put in place by David Nicholson, the then Chief Executive of the NHS, and later Chief Executive of the NHS Commissioning Board which became NHS England, suggested commissioning decisions will be scrutinised. Commissioning groups will also be expected to accept advice from NICE about which treatments they should and should not purchase, in contrast to the original White Paper that proposed greater independence. This advice will be in the form of meeting the quality standards NICE will produce for the NHS, public health and social care.

Foundation trusts will continue to be overseen by Monitor, with a 49 per cent cap on the limit of their permitted private patient activity, and a maximum increase of 5 per cent in such activity in any one year. The application of EU competition law in the NHS is probably constrained, although legal opinion appears to differ with respect to this point as the heated debates over the technicalities of what became known as the 'Section 75' regulations demonstrated. Monitor itself has moved from having a duty to promote competition to preventing anti-competitive behaviour, while at the same time having duties to enable services to be provided in an integrated way that promotes quality and efficiency. It is not clear quite how it will navigate a course through these competing goals. The Secretary of State has retained his or her duty to promote autonomy in NHS institutions, which was central to Lansley's original plan to allow the market to do its work without political interference, but that duty to promote autonomy now has to occur in a context in which there is another duty to promote a comprehensive health service with security of the services it providers. Again, squaring these potentially competing demands is a major challenge.

Finally, the timetable has slowed somewhat, attempting to address concerns that the reorganisation was attempting to achieve too much change, too quickly.

In all, the reorganisation appears to be rather less a radical series of proposals unseen before in the NHS than a continuation and escalation of policy pre-2007. This even appears to be the view of former Labour policy insiders including Julian Le Grand (2011) and Simon Stevens (2010), who, at the time of writing, had just been appointed as Chief Executive of the NHS. In escalating policy pre-2007, however, the reorganisation also creates the potential to go much further than Labour did in terms of privatisation of the NHS (Hunter, 2013a), and occurs at a time when health budgets are under considerable pressure. Such privatisation will be extremely difficult for a future government to undo, even though Labour have promised to repeal the part of the Health and Social Care Act promoting competition. But it will require them to go against the market-based orthodoxy of public reform that they did so much to establish in the 2000s. The original market-based structure of the 2010 White Paper may not have been legislated for in the subsequent Act, but the direction of travel is clear.

In terms of its underpinning programme theory, the final form of the reorganisation can be either seen as a sensible compromise or as a mess. The central components of the changes are a re-emphasis on local dynamic mechanisms, especially those of choice and competition. The 2012 reorganisation re-emphasises choice, giving GP-led commissioners responsibility for purchasing care on the grounds that GPs know which local providers will serve their patients best, while at the same time trying to make those decisions accountable downwards to patients, and upwards to commissioning boards. Competition has been extended to allow public healthcare providers to offer more private services to the NHS marketplace, while at the same time continuing to encourage more non-public provision into healthcare to try and harness competition as a means of improving care.

However, increases in private provision in public providers will have to grow relatively slowly, and the extension of non-public provision will be in an environment not of resource growth, as was the case in the 2000s, but in a more hostile environment, in which budgets are effectively frozen and the NHS attempts to find £20 billion of efficiency savings.

The Cooper debate

As noted in Chapter Five, research from LSE suggested that Labour's reintroduction of the market for care since 2006 had led to lives being saved because of the improvement in mortality rates that appeared to have ensued. The government cited this research in their White Paper as supporting their reorganisation, leading to it becoming central to debates about healthcare reorganisation and evidence assessment, and so it is worth exploring its assumptions and method in some detail, building on the assessment presented in Chapter Five.

Cooper and his colleagues (2011) looked at outcomes data after 2006 and concluded that those areas that, according to their index, had experienced most competition as a result of the changes had experienced improved mortality outcomes in relation to their chosen clinical measure. This research appeared to give credibility to the coalition government plans to increase competition, and is cited in the academic literature as presenting evidence that competition in the NHS led to improved clinical outcomes (Gaynor et al, 2012). However, the findings of this work have proven contentious, and their application to the coalition government's planned reorganisation is far from straightforward.

First, the Cooper et al research effectively treats competition-based reorganisation as having an 'on' date of 2006, measuring its effects from then and attempting to control for other outcomes using statistical analysis ('difference in difference analysis') (Mays, 2011). The problem with this approach is that, as an examination of the history of the NHS shows, passing legislation or putting in place a new policy in healthcare, and successfully implementing it, are two entirely different things. Assuming that from 2006 the NHS was making use of a market mechanism appears to assume that competition and choice were widely taken up at that point, and that this change caused the change. Most patients, according to the national Patient Survey, however, did not even remember being offered a choice, and those who did make a choice usually did it without reference to any data sources (Dixon and Wright, 2008; Dixon, 2009). Given this, assuming that patient choices led to clinical improvements appears a rather big leap, especially when the original research did not even include data concerning referrals to the non-public providers that were meant to be extending choice for them (Pollock et al, 2011). At the same time, as already suggested, qualitative research suggests markets were really not the most significant factor driving managerial thought processes in NHS organisations (Dixon et al, 2010b, p 134).

In all, it seems premature to put any clinical improvements down to increased choice or competition when we have little firm evidence that either were actually happening on the ground (Bevan and Skellern, 2011), and when there was a range of overlapping organisational and policy changes occurring at the same time from the rather hyperactive Labour government (Greener, 2012). Equally, it seems that variables that attempt to measure quality in healthcare are themselves not correlated, meaning that picking one measure (as the Cooper work does) and basing an analysis on that tells us very little (CHE, 2012).

The Cooper research was also conducted in the NHS under Labour's organisational structure, with PCTs doing most of the commissioning, and under a regime in which the market, especially in the period after Gordon Brown became Prime Minister, was being limited by Burnham's expectation that public providers would be 'preferred'. Equally, even if we ignore the problems outlined above, and accept the research at face value in showing that competition between 2006 and 2010 did improve care, then the structures put in place after 2010 by the coalition government are not at all the same. We therefore need new research that shows that the measured improvements have continued beyond that date – especially considering the far tighter budgets for both health and social care after that date.

What Cooper and his collaborators have found is a range of interesting changes in outcomes in that period, even if we can't determine exactly what might have caused them. But suggesting those outcome changes still apply after a significant and costly NHS reorganisation after which the NHS will be required to save £20 billion, when PCTs have been abolished and care commissioning passed to GP-led organisations instead, again appears to be a huge leap in the dark. The NHS, after the coalition reforms, will be an organisation that will have to find new ways of working and forge new relationships in terms of provision and commissioning. We simply don't know how similar any particular locality will be to the NHS in the post-2006 period, and so assuming that research translates from one period to the other in a straightforward way is unrealistic. Expecting any particular governance structure to deliver improvements in healthcare is an act of faith – care is improved by clinicians, managers, other health workers and patients working together, not by the use of markets or hierarchies or networks.

Benefits and costs

In examining the success or otherwise of a particular reorganisation, it is crucial to include both benefits and costs. Without fully considering the costs of introducing a healthcare market, we cannot work out whether that intervention represented good value for money or not. Even if we can find benefits as a result of the adoption of a particular organisational form, we also need to explore whether the cost of that reorganisation might have been better spent simply on employing more clinicians, or improving existing hospital buildings and facilities. If we don't make this comparison, then we aren't including the very significant costs of healthcare reorganisation in our calculations, which are surely crucial in assessing their effectiveness. Indeed, if we factor in the direct and indirect costs of attempting to implement a market for care since the early 2000s, it would be surprising at least if the rather marginal outcomes it appears to have led to could not have been improved on by simply employing more clinicians.

When considering the prospects for the NHS after 2010, we need to pay close attention to the actual institutional arrangements being put in place rather than assuming they more closely resemble any abstract model of ideal type of a market or bureaucracy or anything else, and to work their actual form rather than from an abstract theory or theoretical model. We also need to take care in considering the very considerable costs of reorganising healthcare in England once again, to be aware of the boundary between health and social care, and the problems that partnership working will experience in an era when local authorities are having to work within severely constrained budgets in all areas of the UK.

We can, however, derive some general principles from the research in the 2000s that can inform our understanding of how things may play out in the next few years.

Choice and competition in the NHS

Advocates of the internal or quasi-market in the 1990s argue that the main problem with its lack of success in that decade was not that market mechanisms cannot be made to work well in the NHS, but that there was a lack of competition between hospitals or other healthcare providers (West, 1998). Wider assessments also point to a second significant problem – that patients preferred providers of care that were local to them (Exworthy and Peckham, 2006). Indeed, other researchers suggested that it was questionable whether patients even wanted to make the kind of choices about care referrals they were being offered at all (Fotaki et al, 2005), and others that the use of markets confused the theoretical ideal with a rather more complex reality that it was difficult to argue could work in healthcare (Greener, 2008b). Finally, there was the political problem that large providers of care might be put in a contracting environment driven by market-based incentives, and their financial sustainability be threatened as a result. No Member of Parliament (MP) wants their local hospital to close because of the high-profile public campaigns that will result, no matter how poor-performing it might be.

Labour's 'mixed economy of care', and indeed the coalition reorganisation of the 2010s, represents an attempt to try and deal with several of these problems. These reorganisations attempt to address the problem of there being too little competition for a market to work well by encouraging non-public providers to compete with traditional NHS services, but most private provision of services remains extremely low – at around 2 per cent of the total for care (although this differs in the case of some services, such as in mental health provision, where the figure is much higher) (McLellan, 2012). If competition is meant to be a driving force for improving care, it is not clear how it is meant to happen when non-public provision is so small in the vast majority of treatment areas. For even the less onerous theory of 'contestability' to work, in which competition does not actually have to be in place but just the threat of competition, that threat still has to be real. With non-public provision so small in most areas, neither competition nor contestability are viable, but non-public entry does have the potential to put stretched NHS budgets under increased tension at a time when available funding is static. Equally, because public financing now represents such a large proportion of private healthcare, this means that the private sector is actually far more dependent on NHS contracts than the NHS is on private provision, and so there is a significant imbalance in both power and capacity between the two.

Static budgets

It is also worth stressing that the 2010s are going to be an era of zero or limited budget growth for the NHS, and in which significant efficiency savings will have to be found. If healthcare funding is going to be a zero-sum game (or if we include social care which is funded through local government, then subject to budget reductions), then growth in non-public provision will have to take place at the expense of the availability of funds for public providers. But this will occur in a context in which it is extremely difficult for public hospitals, which often have very high fixed costs, to reduce their activity without running into considerable financial difficulties. Where those providers have made use of PFI deals to rebuild their facilities, the pressures on public providers to achieve high levels of activity will be even greater, and the consequences of them not being able to achieve those levels will be even more likely to lead to financial difficulties.

Public provider failure

Whether public providers of care can or will be allowed to fail through lack of finances is an especially difficult question. Public providers of care are responsible for much of the training of clinicians (although the government is attempting to get non-public providers to take on more of this role), as well as effectively assuring the availability of comprehensive care to the NHS as a whole, as public providers of care tend to be larger, and offer a wider range of services than private providers. When public hospitals in small or medium-size towns become financially bankrupt, there simply is not the capacity from other providers to take up the care of existing patients. Even if the full range of services existed outside the public hospital (which would be unlikely), local people would be unlikely to allow 'their' hospital to close without political protest – and as mentioned above, proposals to even scale back activities at Mid Staffordshire hospital, despite everything that had been written about it in the Francis Report, still led to public demonstrations.

One of the central problems of the coalition government's NHS reorganisation is that they want to extend the market logic, but with no clear plan as to what would happen should a major public hospital or care provider financially fail – indeed, the coalition government has already had to earmark billions in additional funds to allow hospitals with PFI contracts to continue to provide care (Campbell, 2012; Ramesh, 2012). If the new healthcare market is not going to allow organisations that fail financially to go bankrupt, how is using a payment-driven market system meant to drive improvements?

The alternative to allowing public providers to fail has been to bring in management teams from more successful providers, or to try and find hybrid arrangements involving non-public providers such as Circle, who, in 2011, took over the running of Hinchingbrooke Hospital in Cambridge, and so became the first ever non-state provider to run general hospital services in the NHS. The question this approach to addressing failure raises is whether the problems were the result of poor management, or were down to more intractable problems in the local area, such as a lack of adequate care provision in other settings having knock-on effects. If there is a local authority failing to provide adequate social care, this, too, will have an adverse effect on local health services that is beyond the control of NHS managers. It is also possible that specific health services were chosen to inherit budget deficits in the 1990s as a means of rationalising budgetary problems in one location, unaware that they would be held responsible for them in later years. All of these factors mean that we should be cautious of assuming that a particular provider having a financial deficit is necessarily indicative of it doing a bad job. Indeed, if the purchaser–provider split is of questionable value, as the above account suggests it may well be, then the financial result it generates may also be questionable.

Questioning the purchaser–provider split

The evidence supporting using reorganisation based on preserving a purchaser–provider split at all is weak. Despite Labour attempting to put PCT commissioning at the centre of their reorganisations during the 2000s, the House of Commons published a damning report on progress both during the 2000s and 1990s, suggesting that if PCT commissioning 'does not begin to improve soon, after 20 years of costly failure, the purchaser/provider split may need to be abolished' (House of Commons Health Committee, 2009, Conclusions). Given the lack of progress in making the purchaser–provider split work between 1990 and 2010, it does seem strange that it remains the cornerstone of NHS reorganisation in England.

Can it be that it was PCT commissioning, not commissioning per se, that has been the problem? This does not seem to be the case. We know from the 1990s that only the top 10 to 20 per cent of GP fundholders made any real difference in local patterns of care purchasing, with the rest probably not justifying the extra administrative and reorganisation costs involved in their activities (Audit Commision, 1996). If commissioning is to work, it will require a coherent, system-wide approach that aligns policy with commissioning objectives rather than the fragmented and uncoordinated approach put in place in the coalition reorganisation (McCafferty et al, 2012). In July 2013 The King's Fund and Nuffield Trust (Naylor et al, 2013) suggested that there was huge variability in commissioning arrangements and that they were often struggling to secure engagement from GPs, that there was often a lack of clarity about how responsibilities for commissioning were being shared between CCGs and NHS England, and that there were real problems in monitoring the new contractual arrangements, with upheaval and instability still very common.

What about the other problems with attempts in the 1990s to introduce an internal market for care noted above? A major problem is that it still seems that patients prefer care that is local to them. There is some evidence that patients in rural areas are prepared to travel to go to an alternative provider, but this still remains the exception. It is possible, if there was a wider range of providers in urban areas, that patients and GPs would have a greater choice, and so be more likely to refer to high-performing providers, but this in turn depends on GPs and patients using information systems to base their referral choices on, and this is still far from the case. If patients are not choosing or being referred to the highest performing local providers, there seems to be little point in those providers competing with one another to improve their care, and so for competition to be blunted as a mechanism for improvement.

This problem leads us to the issue that what policy-makers often appear to have in mind is an abstract idea that markets improve performance through competition, but with little practical sense of how this can be introduced into healthcare in practice. In realist terms, markets dominate the ideational context within which policy-makers presently formulate their plans for healthcare, but apparently with little reference to the research evidence.

Oligopoly, not competition?

What appears to be the case, without over-generalising, is that there is little competition in most areas of the country – most purchasers of care do not face a large number of alternate providers, but instead an oligopolistic market structure in which there are a small number of providers of care. Within this oligopoly, large public providers are unlikely to be allowed to fail because of the political implications of this, and because they are responsible for much of the comprehensive care provision and clinical training in the local area.

On the purchaser side, GPs and patients do not appear to use what little information there is to make decisions about referrals, and there is little evidence that any form of commissioning we have so far attempted actually makes sufficient difference to demonstrate, in terms of benefits, a net increase when compared to the costs of its introduction. This is not a promising picture, and it is hard to see how we can argue that the extension of choice and competition therefore represents an example of evidence-based policy-making. This leads us to look for other answers as to why there does not appear to be a viable alternative to market-based reorganisation being offered by any of the major political parties in the UK. Perhaps this is a failure of imagination, or perhaps, as the more critical writers in the field suggest, simply a determined and ideologically driven programme to privatise the NHS. Without policy-makers being clear about the goals of their reorganisations, or exactly how they are meant to improve care, it is hard to discount these alternative explanations.

Politicians also have to accept that NHS reorganisation is inherently political. One of the big ideas of the 2010-12 NHS reorganisation was that, by utilising a local dynamic mechanism of improvement, healthcare would become more independent of the government, and so less political as a result. But this is rather naive. The NHS affects all of our lives at some point, spending over £100 billion of tax a year in the process. NHS budgetary decisions can never be the result of a purely technical process.

We want our care to be evidence-based, but there is no single right way to organise healthcare that will make it free from politics. Decisions about how we want our local health services to work can look for general principles from research, but in a democratic society, we need to be arguing about what we want our health services to achieve as well as the best ways of reaching those goals. Surely we want our health services to be more democratically engaged with those they are serving, not less?

Dispelling myths about performance management

Performance management acquired a poor reputation in the NHS in the 2000s, being seen as marred by 'gaming' in which managers and clinicians would conspire to try and make it look as if targets were being met when figures were manipulated and care delivered to try and meet the letter, rather than the spirit, of the performance indicators chosen by government (Mannion et al, 2005; Bevan and Hood, 2006a, 2006b; Hood 2006). As noted in Chapter Four, however, the QOF used in GP surgeries offers an alternative performance management system that appears to have been far more successful.

The QOF appears to have been much more successful because it was based on a set of targets that clinicians regarded as evidence-based, which they had a voice themselves in deciding, and based on practices that could be incorporated into everyday care. In the QOF clinicians had a considerable voice in how they went about achieving the targets set for them, as well as financial incentives at the practice level for achieving their 'points'.

In contrast, hospital-based systems were derived from targets that clinicians regarded as being politically inspired rather than clinically based, which were seen as being imposed on hospitals by government, and which were at an abstract level that day-to-day service decisions did not obviously link to. Clinicians and managers struggled to explain the relevance of targets to staff, leading to them 'gaming' the targets instead, with few incentives for high achievement, but with potential penalties for poor measured performance.

The key point from all of this is that it is possible to use performance management in the NHS, but it needs to be designed rather more according to the principles of the QOF than of those applied in hospitals. This is a challenge, as hospitals offer a wider range of services and operate on a much bigger scale than GP surgeries, but surely it provides a clear role for healthcare managers and clinical leaders to come up with clinically based targets against which they are prepared to be held to account, and to drive improvements on that basis rather than attempting to deal with the abstract, high-level measures presently used, and which often tell us little about the specific services in place in our hospitals.

On coming to power, the coalition government made a point of making it clear they were going to make less use of centralised targets, and, in a market-based system for healthcare, making less use of performance management is clearly logical as the market is meant to provide a strong means for care improvement. However, they have since had to backtrack somewhat from this position, realising that having some element of performance management in place is essential to ensure accountability, especially after the failures at Mid Staffordshire. Taking the more nuanced approach to performance management outlined in this book has the potential to reduce the problems hospitals have experienced with it, while potentially maximising gains.

Patient and public involvement

PPI was another key area of debate in the coalition healthcare organisation. Concerns were raised by those who opposed the bill that there were insufficient checks and balances on CCGs, a concern that appears to have been acknowledged in amendments so that there are now statutory duties for consultation on commissioning, and on the establishment of commissioning groups. The devil, however, once again, will be in the detail. Some localities may want to embrace the spirit of greater public involvement in commissioning, and so seek opportunities to find ways to make commissioning more locally accountable and responsive to local need. Other areas, however, may be more tokenistic. As noted above, the NHS does not generally have a strong record on achieving deep public involvement in decision-making, even if some areas have been a beacon for its achievement and improvement (Wistow, 2001; Callaghan and Wistow, 2006a, 2006b). The evidence appears to suggest that the public want deep and ongoing opportunities for significant involvement in healthcare decision-making, but whether these opportunities will be made available seems doubtful.

The Francis Report, performance management and patient and public involvement

The Francis Report (2013), which investigated the care failures at Mid Staffordshire Hospital in the late 2000s, offers us a range of crucial insights into the workings of performance management systems and PPI organisations in the NHS, and so is worth reflecting on, as well as having the potential to shape the coalition government's health policy.

Francis found, across a range of inquiries (Francis, 2010, 2013), that the appalling care failings at Mid Staffordshire were due to a systemic failure of care provision within the NHS. Poor care became systemic in some areas of the hospital, and where it was reported to both senior managers at the trust, and to managers in other healthcare organisations, they did not act on those reports. There are even cases of senior managers dismissing such reports or attempting to counter-brief local media that the dreadful stories emerging about patient neglect were unfounded.

What is particularly dreadful is that poor care at Mid Staffordshire does not appear to have been a clustering of problems appearing at different times and places, but an everyday occurrence. Furthermore, the report asserts that Mid Staffordshire is unlikely to be an isolated case. The importance of the findings lies not only in highlighting failings and reasons for those failings at a particular trust, but also in drawing attention to failings that may be happening elsewhere in the NHS.

At the same time as the failings at Mid Staffordshire, the government had put in place their performance management system that was meant to pick up such problems, a system of regulation that was meant to mean care failings would be investigated, and patient and public representative organisations in place that were meant to challenge hospital management with reports of problems. How on earth did such care failure occur despite all of this?

Francis suggests in his report that the failures at Mid Staffordshire were systemic and cultural – even though the problems were known by those who had the power to deal with them, managers were too busy chasing process-based targets and trying to achieve 'financial balance' than to look after patients well, and when patients and the public raised concerns, the trust did not act on their concerns. As such, Mid Staffordshire was a failure both of the performance management system and of PPI – of both central control and local dynamic mechanisms.

Francis suggests that what the NHS needs is to set clearly defined basic care standards that trusts must adhere to, and that staff who provide care below that standard, or even allow others to do so, should face disciplinary or even legal punishment. His report suggests that those in charge of health services must show stronger leadership, and that compassionate patient care needs to be the focus of the NHS again.

Based on the research reviewed here, Francis' recommendations in relation to care standards, with all due respect to the extraordinary work he did in gathering the deeply affecting evidence of patients and the public and the care he showed in compiling his report, seem unlikely to work. Setting central standards which healthcare professionals do not have a say in, do not regard as being based on best practice as opposed to basic standards, and which do not directly relate to their everyday practice, are what made performance management systems dysfunctional in the 2000s. Moreover, despite advocating the need for widespread culture change, Francis displayed only a weak understanding of culture in complex healthcare contexts (Davies and Mannion, 2013, p 3), not comprehending the considerable cultural diversity present in any NHS organisation and the 'varying degrees of autonomy and empowerment of different players' in healthcare organisations as a result.

Where Francis is correct is the need for 'impact assessment' of structural changes to the NHS, setting out a comprehensive set of questions that policy-makers should answer before putting in place changes that draw attention to the political context within which the NHS operates, and which have the potential to inform the likely effects of the introduction of new policies. Given the furore over and lengthy debate resulting from the coalition's Health and Social Care Bill, it is surely the case that an adequate impact assessment, had it been carried out openly and transparently, would have led to the government thinking again.

Where Francis is also correct is the real need for the stronger representation of voices, especially when it comes to patients, to speak against dominant interests and to challenge poor care practices. Sadly, it is hard to see how Healthwatch can meet this brief, given its consumer-based role, and the loss of learning from previous patient representative organisations that has occurred.

In keeping with Francis' diagnosis, what research evidence suggests has a better chance of working is for multidisciplinary care teams to be made responsible for improving the care under their control, with performance standards set against clinically led benchmarks, and with those staff undergoing management development programmes to work together better and to develop respect for one another's professional skills. Such teams can be held accountable should care not reach the needed level, as well as having a basis for arguing for additional resources, should they be needed, by benchmarking their own resource usage against comparable teams elsewhere. These suggestions also go very much with the grain of the Keogh review into the quality of care and treatment in NHS hospitals (Keogh, 2013), and the Berwick review of the changes to patient safety needed after Mid Staffordshire (Berwick, 2013), with the latter especially stressing the importance of team learning, simple and clear supervisory systems that avoid the diffusion of responsibility, and that recourse to the criminal sanctions proposed by Francis be extremely rare.

It is also worth reflecting whether it even makes any sense to talk about 'compassionate care', as Francis does. As Mol (2008) makes clear, the 'logic of care' inherently contains compassion – it would be an oxymoron to talk about 'uncompassionate care'. Care in the NHS in the contemporary world is inherently complex and multidisciplinary, but for it to be 'care', it has to have compassion, otherwise it is something else. But care requires time and patience and an acceptance that it is a shared enterprise between patient and clinician (and family and friends), and it is hard to see how market-based dynamics, which necessarily have to include limits to what care can be provided in order for it to be commodified, can be made to fit within a framework where care is meant to be at the centre. The role of leadership in this process is key in setting a context within which the quality of care is uppermost, where patients have a voice in speaking out against poor practice, and where staff are able to bring attention to failings without fear of reprisals. Perhaps the biggest lesson from Mid Staffordshire is that, without strong leadership, clinicians' attention can be taken away from care through poor performance measures, and on to an over-concern with financial balance instead.

The failure of PPI mechanisms at Mid Staffordshire, given the research findings above, does not come as a surprise. The repeated reorganisation of PPI organisations during the 2000s led to a loss of experienced staff and to a lack of continuity that was not conducive to the serious, engaged and challenging work of holding those providing poor care to account. It is crucial that the NHS does better in the future, but a starting point is consolidating existing organisations responsible for PPI rather than reorganising them again. Patients and the public need a strong engaged voice in healthcare, and organisations providing care in the NHS, both public and non-public, need clear mechanisms by which they are held to account by their local communities, with public concerns about the quality and standard of care taken seriously not only by specific providers of care, but also by those responsible for regulating them.

The private finance initiative

Finally, PFI is a becoming significant problem whose financial consequences are becoming widely felt within the NHS. The PFI contracts that were signed in the resource-richer times of the 2000s to build new hospitals and GP surgeries are now, under increased budgetary pressures and potentially greater competition, much less affordable. In 2012, the Secretary of State made £1.5 billion available to 'bail out' some hospital trusts that could not meet their PFI payments (Campbell, 2012). In late 2012, the most poorly paid staff at Mid Yorkshire Hospital Trust were facing regrading exercises to try and save money so that the trust could find ways of paying its PFI maintenance payments, and was far from alone in having to find such savings. Many hospital trusts, unable to pay the PFI bills that they now face, are trying to find ways of buying out their contracts, but this in turn will involve significant fundraising and close cooperation with local government in order to make it possible.

If hospitals (and GP surgeries) are going to be judged on the basis of whether they are able to show they are, within the constraints of PbR, financially viable, they will have to find ways of meeting the PFI maintenance payments they have signed up for. However, PFI contracts appear to have generated over-generous returns for the private partners, due in part to the naivety of the representatives of NHS organisations who entered into complex contracting processes with far more experienced private sector partners, and in part due to the poor design of the PFI process itself (Asenova and Beck, 2003, 2010), which failed to standardise contracts or offer opportunities for learning and improvement in the contracting process. It was politicians who designed a contracting process that created these problems, making public infrastructure investment almost unavailable by any other means. It is surely therefore for politicians to take responsibility for fixing it.

PFI is a problem that is not going to go away for those who have signed its agreements. The case for the government intervening and renegotiating the contracts en masse appears to be compelling. The argument against this contract renegotiation is that it would lead to private companies not generating the profits that their signed contracts entitled them to, and so to firms not wanting to contract with the government in the future. However, in the cases of well-publicised rail franchise failures, for example, private companies appear to have reneged on agreements with few penalties attached, and without losing the ability to tender for government contracts again. The most prestigious case of private failure occurred where security firm G4S fell well short of their contracted duties weeks before the Olympics, and so the armed forces had to be drafted in to fill the gap, but without G4S losing their right to tender for government work in the future.

It is very honourable that the government might wish to ensure that PFI contracts are paid for in full, but where those contracts have led to manifestly above-market levels of reward, and to the need for huge bail-outs in order for cash-strapped hospitals to continue to operate, then it is surely time to look again at the long-term commitments NHS organisations have undertaken.

Equally, the problems with PFI, combined with the problems at Mid Staffordshire, pose deep questions about whether healthcare organisations ought to be run as businesses in competitive marketplaces, contracting with private sector organisations to construct their buildings and maintain their wards. We are not suggesting that healthcare organisations be run without regard to budgets, or that there is no room for better management within them – we hope the recommendations we have made above make that clear. However, we would surely prefer our healthcare organisations to spend their energy focused on providing the best possible care than negotiating building contracts, competing with other healthcare organisations, and having to cut the pay of their most poorly paid staff to pay for maintenance contracts that they can no longer afford.

Comparing healthcare reorganisation in England, Scotland, Wales and Northern Ireland

A central part of the realist method is to make clear that context matters. In the UK, this is perhaps most clear in the diverging approach to healthcare policy and reorganisation evident in each of the four countries within it since the introduction of political devolution in 1999.

In general terms, since 1999 England has tended to move towards a model in which first performance management was put in place, and then, from the middle of the 2000s, there has been an emphasis on competition to attempt to drive improvements. The NHS in England is also undergoing a significant reorganisation, as noted above, in which GP-led commissioning groups have assumed the role of commissioning from PCTs, and with the encouragement of an increase in non-public provision to drive competitive processes. Wales and Scotland have chosen to go down distinctly different paths, with Scotland putting in place a more integrated health system with no purchaser–provider split, no contracting for care between providers and commissioners, and a commitment to the 1999 Royal Commission on Long-Term Care of putting in place free personal care for older people (which England and Wales have not adopted). Scotland's health service structures have broadly remained unchanged since 2004. Wales, like Scotland, has emphasised partnership working rather than competition, with little or no role for the private sector in the delivery of care, but has seen some reorganisation in 2009 in the form of a reduction in the number of local health boards, but with all major parties committed to avoiding further reorganisations. Hunter (2013b, p 2) goes further in suggesting that the Scottish health and healthcare system is attempting to break with the Anglo-Saxon tradition and put in place an 'ethos marked by collectivism, reciprocity and a commitment to public services.' Greer and Trench (2008) pithily summarise the differences as England – 'markets and management', Scotland – 'medical profession and cooperation', Wales – 'localism and wider public health' and

Northern Ireland – 'permissive managerialism'. Northern Ireland has at least in theory joint commissioning of health and social care in a structure that includes a purchaser–provider split, but with an emphasis on consultation and cooperation.

The process of devolution, and the ensuing policy divergence outlined above, suggests the possibility of comparison and learning between the four healthcare systems to try and establish which approach (markets, choice and competition in England, a greater emphasis on retaining and strengthening the public interest and partnership working in Scotland and Wales) appears to work the best. Indeed, it has become commonplace to refer to devolution as representing a 'natural experiment' from which we can learn (Propper et al, 2010). From a realist perspective, devolution represents an opportunity for learning, but is some distance from being a natural experiment. For a natural experiment to be in place, we would have to be starting in each healthcare system from a similar position, to be able to put in place controls so we were sure which interventions were being introduced in each system and what their effects were, and to be able to be sure about what the causal links were that led to improved (or worse performance) in each case. Instead, however, there are definite limits on the extent to which we can understand each of the healthcare systems out of their immediate contexts as they are all complex, adaptive systems in their own right. What this means is that we have to be extremely careful in making claims for, and generalisations between, the four health systems in the UK – the four countries had different starting points in terms of their health outcomes, have considerable differences in health outcomes within their own boundaries, and reorganisations have not been implemented uniformly in each country, especially when compared with the (from a policy change perspective) hyperactive England.

In many respects it would make more sense, from a realist perspective, to be comparing specific regions with similar characteristics in each of the countries in depth in order to generate programme theories rather than to attempt broad-brush country-level comparisons that often conceal as much as they reveal. This approach is also favoured by the Nuffield Trust that has used the North East of England to compare with the other devolved nations on similar grounds (Connolly et al, 2010). However, it does make sense to try and compare health systems across the four countries and to try and work out what each country can learn from the others.

A significant problem faced by country-based comparisons is that attempts to compare the results of different reorganisations in each of the different countries have been dogged by the data collected not being in a form that is easily comparable (Blackman et al, 2010; Wilson, 2011).

Despite all of these caveats, we can see some general trends in comparisons between the four countries that are worth exploring in more depth.

Performance management

First, if we compare Wales, Scotland and England in terms of the healthcare system's use of performance management, we can generate some useful learning for policy and practice. England was the first to put in place a target-driven performance management system, outlining its form in the 2000 NHS Plan (Secretary of State for Health, 2000), and then introducing tables of performance against them a year later (DH, 2001c). England was the only one of the devolved countries to explicitly link increased funding with improved measured performance (Connolly et al, 2010). As noted above, the use of targets has brought considerable problems in terms of 'gaming' within hospitals especially, and there are allegations that their use has distorted clinical priorities in favour of chasing easily measurable outcomes such as waiting times (Bevan and Hood, 2006b; Harrington et al, 2009; Smith et al, 2009). At the same time as these league tables were compiled, managerial performance was often assessed in terms of managers' ability to meet such targets, and short-term contracts meant that a regime of 'targets and terror' (Bevan and Hood, 2006b) was instigated under the Labour government. At the same time as these concerns, however, waiting times 'duly fell, sharply and steadily' (Timmins, 2013, p 13), and waiting times fell faster in England than they did in any of the other three countries (Andrews and Martin, 2010). The other three countries introduced their own forms of performance management, although none as robust as England's in linking measurable achievement against outcomes with success or as 'draconian' in threatening chief executives' jobs if targets were repeatedly missed (Timmins, 2013). The differences in both the way targets have been introduced and the way that organisations have been assessed in their performance against them reveal some key differences.

In performance managing health inequalities in the 2000s, targets in England focused on reducing social class differences in infant mortality and area-based life expectancy by 10 per cent, while Scotland focused on health improvement rather than inequality targets, and Wales put in place health inequality targets to produce a faster rate of improvement with the national average for the most deprived groups. In addition, there were different timescales for meeting targets in the different countries – Scotland had a timescale of 2008, England 2010 and Wales 2020 (Blackman et al, 2006, 2010). This reflects both differences in approach to health policy, as seen above in the quotation from Greer and Trench, and also a recognition by Welsh and Scottish governments that their public health needs (that is, to improve life expectancy for the general population) and therefore priorities were different from England. However, the picture was further complicated by a shifting political climate. In Wales in particular the initial lack of concern over targets and a focus on underlying determinants of health inequalities changed after the removal of Jane Hutt as Health Minister for the Welsh Assembly Government in 2005 and in the face of considerable media and political pressure to a focus on cutting long hospital waiting lists (Harrington et al, 2009; Smith et al, 2009).

Given that performance management is with us, in all four countries, and is likely to stay, it is surely important that we do the best job we can, which brings increased urgency to the recommendations outlined above in terms of what performance management in hospitals can usefully learn from the experience of the introduction of the QOF in GP surgeries. However, it really is worth stressing that a great deal more research needs to be carried out in this area.

Integrated care

A second area where some learning could occur is when comparing the four countries' different approaches to integrating care. Although a first difficultly is definitional – as Timmins (2013, p 17) reminds us, care can be integrated (as a starting point) between primary and secondary (and tertiary) settings, between health and social care, between health and community care, and between physical and mental care – it does appear that having a single managerial body attempting to manage the integration of primary and secondary care, as in Scotland, Wales and Northern Ireland, seems to improve things significantly.

What does seem to make a difference in integrating care more generally is some degree of stability in terms of organisational arrangements (Timmins, 2013, p 17). Again, the contrast between Scotland and the hyperactive England comes to mind, and it is surely no coincidence that the World Health Organization (WHO), for example, attributes a great deal of Scotland's success in improving healthcare outcomes to its organisational and political stability over the last decade (Steel and Cyclus, 2012), suggesting that stability is an important factor not only for integrated care, but also for the delivery of care more generally.

Competition and markets

There are clearly significant differences between the four countries in terms of their use of the purchaser–provider split. In England, Labour reinstated a market for care in the mid-2000s which the coalition government extended in its healthcare reorganisation, but with Scotland and Wales not following suit, and although Northern Ireland has a purchaser–provider split, the emphasis appears to be far more on collaboration than the competition which is meant to drive health service improvement in England. The major problem in comparing data concerning the market is disentangling its effects from all the other reorganisations in England at the same time (Mays and Dixon, 2011), and also the lack of data comparing the costs of the market-based reorganisation against any benefits that might have accrued. It appears to be the case that 'politicians from Scotland, Wales and Northern Ireland would, in the main, argue that they have learnt from the English experience, not to adopt such an approach' (Timmins, 2013, p 13).

The use of competition in healthcare poses significant research challenges because of the difficulty of disentangling causal effects, and also because competition-based policies have themselves continually changed since their full introduction into the NHS in England in about 2006, with the coalition government making the biggest change in moving commissioning from PCTs (now abolished) to CCGs, and with local adaptation of the centrally set framework making even inside-England comparisons difficult to achieve (Dixon and Jones, 2011).

Inputs and outputs

A final point is that there are different rates of expenditure and staffing in the four countries. In general, England (based on 2006 figures) has the lowest rates of expenditure per capita, as well as the lowest rates of nurses, hospital medical and dental staff; Scotland tends to have the highest. Northern Ireland has the highest rates per capita of management and support staff, with England again being the lowest on those measures (Connolly et al, 2010). It therefore seems that English healthcare is comparatively efficient (although such comparisons, as noted, are fraught with difficulty due to finding comparable data and because of the different contextual settings), but there are questions as to whether the more collaborative forms of organisation in the other three nations will produce longer-term benefits or might be better at generating improvements in other areas such as public engagement (Andrews and Martin, 2010).

Comparing the four countries

As we hope we have made clear, comparisons between the four countries over the 2000s are fraught with problems while also providing useful insights and raising questions about the best approach to improving health and healthcare. However, it does seem reasonable to say that performance management, despite its problems, has become a central feature of healthcare organisation across the four countries of the UK, that putting in place greater stability in organisational arrangements is likely to lead to improvements in health outcomes (a feature that has been particularly apparent in Scotland), and that the use of competition and markets remains contentious, with little strong data supporting their current use in England, especially in terms of comparing the costs of introducing and extending competition against what appear to be the relatively small improvements that might have accrued as a result.

What is very apparent is that, as health has become a politically devolved responsibility in Wales, Scotland and Northern Ireland, this has led to greater discretion in health policy, especially in terms of expenditure. It is also the case that the devolved nations, especially Scotland, have led the way in terms of public health innovations such as smoking bans in public buildings and minimum alcohol unit pricing.

In England, government promises to protect health budgets have tended to conceal the significant reductions in social services expenditure since 2010, which will have fallen by a quarter by 2014, and so will surely lead to problems in integration between health and community health services. Wales, in contrast, will see a 10 per cent fall in NHS spending by 2014, which will be the largest reduction in its history, but with social services falling by around 4 per cent, putting the system as a whole under considerable strain. Scotland has seen a fall of around 4 per cent in healthcare spending, and Northern Ireland has seen a reduction of around 2 per cent, which would seem to indicate health services are coming under pressure, but not to the same extent as in Wales. In an era of austerity, the apparently inexorable post-war rise in healthcare expenditure has come to an end in all four countries, putting all four systems under different degrees of pressure, the results of which may take years for us to uncover.

Conclusion

The prospects for NHS reform after 2010 appear rather bleak. The coalition's health reorganisation was based on market-based principles that appear to have little support in research, and it is surely time to look again at whether the purchaser–provider split is a sensible basis for organising healthcare. The split persists only in England, and whereas we certainly need more research comparing system performance with Scotland and Wales specifically, it does not seem likely that the costs involved in maintaining the market in England can exceed the limited benefits that seem to accrue from it. Scotland in particular has eschewed wholesale structural and organisational change in its health services, also choosing not to go down the path of market-based organisation, preferring not to extend competition or increase patient choice. As a result, it has an integrated system of healthcare that presents a real alternative to the English, marketised model, and which has made considerable progress in terms of population health and the quality and effectiveness of care (Steel and Cyclus, 2012). There are considerable problems in comparing outcomes in Scotland with those of England as Scotland started at such a disadvantage at the beginning of the 2000s, but it is important to note that the European Health Observatory put much of its success down to 'a relative lack of organisational turbulence' that has 'provided a strong launching pad for achieving beneficial change' (Steel and Cyclus, 2012, p xxi). The contrast with England in this regard is stark.

Performance management has acquired a terrible reputation in hospital organisation, but this is perhaps more due to the rather clumsy way it was introduced and implemented in the 2000s than because the idea itself is flawed. The success of the QOF in changing GP behaviour shows that a flexible and evidence-based approach to performance management can work, but it will require policy-makers to rethink their approach to setting targets, and for managers and clinicians to behave in more collaborative ways to make sure the approach can work in hospitals.

The PPI mechanisms put in place by the coalition government can work in any number of ways, depending on particular local circumstances and how seriously their healthcare organisations treat the processes they put in place for achieving their goals. However, a sensible default position might be one of scepticism towards potential success – achieving meaningful participation is a time-consuming and challenging process, and there is little to suggest that the new healthcare organisations have the time, resources or expertise to achieve it. Finally, PFI represents a huge albatross threatening the viability of the healthcare organisations that signed contracts in the 2000s. Unless the government is prepared to get involved in renegotiating the deals across the board, it is hard to see how the organisations affected can expect to face anything except repeated financial failures in the future.

We recommend that policy-makers stop looking for solutions in endlessly reorganising the NHS, and instead understand that improving healthcare requires putting in place some research-based principles and a great deal of hard work in implementation. This is the opposite of the way in which health policy is usually prosecuted – with a great deal of time and effort going into presenting and negotiating complex organisational structures, but little attempt being made in actually implementing them. This is because policy-makers have the most control over the policy-making process, and the least over implementation, but no great idea held by policy-makers, no matter how much it has the potential to change healthcare for the better, will lead to anything unless it is implemented successfully, and this requires policy-makers to work with those who actually provide care. The 2010-12 reorganisation alienated so many of those working in the NHS that it has almost created vested interests in the organisation not succeeding.

Following the principles outlined here, which are far less contentious but have a genuine chance of making a difference, should change the focus from policy-making towards the hard business of making healthcare better. It requires close cooperation between policy-makers and those working in the health services, and also an acceptance that there really are no magic answers.

Reflecting back on NHS reorganisation: revisiting the 'shared version' in 2013

This book began by using a framework put together by Harrison, Hunter and Pollitt that was a reasonable descriptive device for considering health politics during the 1980s, the 'shared version'. We can now update this device to consider the current situation in 2013.

In 2013 in England, although not elsewhere in the UK, we have become accustomed to the idea of wide-ranging, significant healthcare reorganisation in a way that seemed unimaginable in the 1980s. With hindsight, the first internal market reorganisation in the early 1990s was instrumental in this regard in that it was the first time the government put in place a significant structural reorganisation without consulting doctors, and in face of their opposition. Even if the first internal market led, in the end, to much less change than might have first appeared, its politics changed subsequent healthcare reorganisations in that governments have not always felt obliged to consult or work with doctors in the way they felt obliged to in the 1970s. Labour's healthcare reorganisations began with extensive consultations in 1997 and particularly in 2000, during the formulation of the NHS Plan, but as market-based changes were reintroduced, consultations became less widespread, and by the time of the 2010 reorganisation, the coalition government, as with the first internal market reforms, introduced their changes in the face of considerable opposition from all quarters, not just the medical profession.

Central government has therefore become much stronger in terms of health politics, and so able to act without consulting or working with health professionals to a much greater extent in policy-making. This doesn't mean, however, that the government can control the implementation of its policy ideas. The increased strength of the government in policy-making is in some ways justified – it did sometimes appear in the 1990s as if medical regulatory bodies such as the General Medical Council were more interested in protecting their members than the public (Sandford, 2001). In some areas, the government has made significant inroads into confronting medical power. Clinical governance has led to doctors in particular being held far more to account than ever before, and the coalition government's proposals over medical regulation, which requires doctors to go through far stronger reaccreditation processes than possibly anywhere else in the world, show that the government has become far more daring in challenging clinical power than at any other period. However, whether this approach will lead to real change on the ground is another question. The government requires the active cooperation of those providing care to make any reorganisation work, and alienating them by introducing changes many clinicians regard as badly thought out, or are even opposed to, is unlikely to achieve such cooperation. Doctors in particular may have lost their veto over policy, but their engagement and support is still essential and required for successful policy implementation – a message the government may have forgotten or even ignored.

Health services organisations are still, for the most part, rather introverted in their outlook. They are large, bureaucratic entities that have their own cultures (and sub-cultures), and it is possible, in many cases, for people to spend their entire careers working within them, oblivious to the events and pressures around them. What has changed, however, is that hospitals especially are now under far greater pressure to balance their books, to show they are achieving good levels of performance, and even to find ways of competing with new entrants in their local health economies. They also have to show how they are responding and adapting to changes in healthcare needs and population changes in respect of a growing elderly population with co-morbidities, many of whom do not require hospital care either for lengthy periods or at all, but which demands effective integration across primary, secondary and tertiary care as well as social care. Healthcare managers have to work within budgets and face performance targets which, should they not be met, could lead to them losing their jobs – in particular, managers responsible for delivering performance targets. In an era where healthcare budgets are no longer growing in real terms, and more organisations are attempting to compete for healthcare contracts, managers have to find ways of at least retaining their organisations' market shares and so not suffering real falls in the resources available to them. And in organisations with PFI contracts of one kind or another, real savings have to be found simply to make such agreements, signed in a period of year-on-year budget increases, affordable in a time when budgets may even be falling. Managerial roles are better paid, and have higher status than in previous decades, but they also carry much higher risks.

Despite all of the rhetoric about choice and healthcare consumerism, patients and patient representative groups are still weak players in health politics – the 'repressed interests' in Alford's classic taxonomy of structural interests in healthcare systems (Alford 1975). It can still be difficult to get the NHS to respond quickly and effectively to patient complaints (Clwyd and Hart, 2013), and the continual reorganisation of public and patient representative bodies has left them in a situation where they struggle to make an impact in driving up care standards or addressing significant problems. This is not helped by the increasing complexity of healthcare provision, which now has to work across not only organisational boundaries within the NHS, which has always been difficult enough, but across public/non-public boundaries, and engaging increasing numbers of different kinds of providers of care. Care has become increasingly fragmented as it takes place across a wider and wider range of different organisations, leading to the risk that problems are not being addressed and dealt with, as blame too becomes spread, with no one willing to take responsibility or providing integrated care. These changes are summarised in Table 6.1 below.

The NHS of 2013 is a very different one from that which existed in the 1980s, but the healthcare system has been transformed to reveal a whole range of new challenges in addition to some that remain largely unresolved.

Table 6.1: The 'shared version' of health politics in the 1980s and 2013

Shared version feature	1980s	2013
Incrementalism	Changes tend to be slow, and narrow in scope	Changes now wide-ranging, introduced on short timescales
Partisan mutual adjustment	No one actor or institution is able to dominate	Government has become much stronger
Medical profession have veto power	Doctor representative bodies are able to prevent policy changes that might adversely affect doctors in the NHS	Doctors no longer able to veto policy, but still have significant control over implementation
Lay health authority members in a weak position compared to doctors or managers	Health services are run with little reference to external pressures or controls – 'introversion'	Health services still introverted, but under considerable financial, performance and competitive pressures
Health consumer groups are weak	Health consumer groups have become more concentrated, but still exert relatively little power over decision-making processes	Health consumer groups still weak. Individual complaints still poorly dealt with
The 'centre' has little operational control over implementation, but does have control over resource allocation and distribution	Central government has little control and little information about how health services are run, but does control the overall budget and how it is distributed regionally	Central government has much greater control and information, but increasingly taking less responsibility – decentralisation of blame
Health authority managers are largely 'reactive'	Managerial roles tend to be about fire-fighting, diplomacy, conflict-avoidance and consensus-seeking	Managerial roles are more high status, but there is a threat of sacking in poorly performing organisations and concern that the financial balance is the main focus
Complexity of system contributes to inertia	The vast size and complexity of health services combined with entrenched interest groups makes change very difficult	Complexity is increased as services become more fragmented across public–private boundaries
Durable political consensus	No government has challenged the 'double bed' relationship between the state and the medical profession (see above), and the NHS continues to be popular and supported by the public	Government has challenged the 'double bed' relationship and is now able to enact significant reorganisation in the face of medical opposition and despite public opposition

The political context at the end of 2013 is one in which the government has expended a great deal of political capital in getting the Health and Social Care Bill into place in the face of concerted opposition, but with the resulting Act requiring a great deal of hard work to implement. This is not only because of its somewhat contradictory nature – being the result of compromise and so much amendment – but also because so many clinicians have been alienated during the introduction of the Bill, because reorganising commissioning has resulted in a great deal of disruption and because the NHS has had to go through the reorganisation at a time when it has also faced significant budgetary pressures. The political environment is not a positive one – at the time of writing Labour are still promising to repeal the Health and Social Care Act if they form the next government, although it is not entirely clear what they might put in its place. However, this is to create uncertainty at a time when those within the NHS are already struggling to make the reorganisation work.

Ideationally, the position is also somewhat contradictory. Despite the lack of evidence that the benefits from market-based reforms exceed their now significant costs, and the availability of alternative models in other parts of the UK, extending choice and competition remain the cornerstone of the main political parties' approach to healthcare organisation in England. The appointment of Simon Stevens, who was the main government adviser at the time of Labour's reintroduction of the healthcare market in the 2000s, as the incoming Chief Executive of the NHS, suggests that this emphasis is not likely to change. It seems as if health policy is dominated by a mindset that choice and competition are the only possible way forward, regardless of the costs of previous reorganisations based on those principles.

The problems experienced by performance management policies, which we might regard as the main alternative to choice and competition, during the 2000s partially account for the dominance of market-based approaches. But this is not the whole story – health policy takes place in a context where the common sense of policy-makers has been based on the derogation of professionalism and of public services, with entrepreneurship, the private sector and not-for-profits being celebrated instead. Even if we put to one side claims that the NHS is being privatised or dismantled – and there are grounds for having legitimate concerns that this is the case – then the often blind faith placed in non-public provision appears extraordinary from an evidence-based perspective, at a time when there have been care scandals in private social care homes, and well-publicised mis-selling and misrepresentation of health services in private provision-dominated areas such as cosmetic surgery. It is certainly the case that the publicly provided NHS has had to confront significant failures in care, but to imagine that greater non-public provision would have prevented these failings is to ignore the simple truth that bad care is bad care, regardless of which sector produces it, and to cling to a naive belief that choice and competition can act as a means of preventing it from occurring.

The final chapter considers the use of evidence in health reorganisation and what alternative options exist in place of the current healthcare reorganisation.

SEVEN

Conclusion

> But rather than looking – again – for a structural answer that will work the same way everywhere right across the country, maybe it's time for more emergent models, more experimentation, and more diversity. (Stevens, 2011)

Introduction

In July 2013, the government withdrew its plans to put in place minimum unit alcohol pricing and plain tobacco packaging in England on the grounds that there was insufficient evidence to support these proposals, and despite Scotland already progressing such ideas. As such, three years after the general election of 2010, the government was still claiming that its approach to healthcare was evidence-based, albeit in the face of (in relation to these plans at least) considerable scepticism from the media and public.

This chapter considers what it means to be concerned about evidence and health reorganisation, and restates the book's central ideas and findings.

Evidence and policy

The ideal model of the link between evidence and policy has the former informing the latter, with policy then being carefully evaluated before creating new evidence on which new policy is based, in a virtuous circle stretching off into the future. But we know this doesn't happen. Policy-makers can come with their own ideas, evidence can be more equivocal or technical than policy-makers might like, and the best of intentions on both sides may be derailed by miscommunication and the urgency of problems of the day taking priority over a more careful, reflective approach. Health policy, be it at the local or national level, often appears to be as much about the influence and importance of particular individuals over the process as their mastery of research evidence (Oliver et al, 2012).

Equally, assuming that evidence-gathering and synthesis is a purely technical process that can produce unequivocal answers that are guaranteed to work is both to deny human agency and to raise the expectations of policy-makers and the public to a level that cannot possibly be met. Researchers have an obligation to be measured and cautious in their recommendations, as well as being aware of the limitations of their own work. Making recommendations for policy is too important to not contain caveats and make clear the need for contextualisations. If this frustrates policy-makers, who might want simple answers about 'what works', then perhaps the fault lies with those seeking simple answers to complex problems rather than with researchers attempting to better understand the world. At the same time, however, researchers have a responsibility to present their findings in a way that policy-makers can have the best chance of understanding. They need to bear in mind Einstein's aphorism that everything should be made as simple as possible – but no simpler.

Realist approach to healthcare evidence

The approach adopted in this book has been to take a realistic, theory-driven view of evidence. Rather than believing there are simple answers to the complex and 'wicked' problems of healthcare organisation that can be derived by running regressions or undertaking costly randomised controlled trials (RCTs), and which will work universally across the diverse range of healthcare settings, we have argued that instead we need to pay far closer attention to the role of context in healthcare research, and to accept that there may be no single or right answers to healthcare reform.

We are not powerless to make health services better, however – there does seem to be evidence that some ways of organising healthcare have a better chance of succeeding than others. Policy-makers who put healthcare organisations through continual reorganisations are wasting public money on a massive scale and chasing often unachievable goals – or even not making the goals of their reorganisations clear in the first place. To do this is to avoid the sheer hard work of trying to finding ways of supporting clinicians and other healthcare professionals in making care better, and supporting patients and the public in engaging in the running of their local health services to make them more accountable. Things can be made better, but to expect it to happen overnight as a consequence of the introduction of markets or bureaucracies or any other organisational form is simply not going to happen.

Crucially, it is important to recognise that improving healthcare organisations requires a more careful, nuanced and contextual use of research. Careful investigations, both quantitative and qualitative, are required that take full account of the different contexts healthcare organisations are working within, and which accept that we are not dealing with closed systems where we can put in place laboratory controls and isolate the effects of different policy interventions, but instead with open, messy, complex systems that have fuzzy boundaries and are inhabited by people with choices.

We need to accept that researching healthcare organisations requires work that treats them not as simple machines, where the effects of introducing particular practices can be readily measured and assessed, and where they seem to make a positive difference, to be rolled out to the rest of the NHS in an unproblematic way. Instead, investigations should not assume any intervention has been uniform in application or in its context. We need research that can put together theories about what seems to work best (and what does not), and also to develop explanations of how context affects the way things work out. We can then begin to try and establish explanations of health reorganisation, and principles by which we achieve the best chance of building on those explanations to proceed in an evidence-informed way.

Evidence can never tell us whether a particular healthcare reorganisation will work. It has to be more careful and measured. Contexts change, mechanisms will not be introduced in the same way everywhere, and outcomes may be difficult to measure.

Some alternative principles for more successful healthcare reorganisation

Despite the government's claims that the present health reorganisation in England is based on evidence (and the global trend towards using market mechanisms to try and improve healthcare), we believe that the market-based principles on which they are based are not supported either theoretically or empirically.

What healthcare is (and is not)

Planning and providing healthcare is not the same thing as putting together a supply chain for a retail store – it requires professionals who have years of training and massive investments in complex technologies, the use of which often allow little or no margin for error without serious consequences for patients. Equally, patients are not consumers of health. They often lack the expertise to make the best choices for themselves. This is not a matter of patronising people – clinicians have years of training in order to diagnose and treat patients, and it is unrealistic to expect the public to acquire complex understandings of illnesses and injuries so they can make choices for themselves without investing considerable time and money in systems that can support them in doing so. Excellent healthcare is about partnerships between clinicians and patients, and getting health services to work in a coordinated and caring manner. No governance or organisational form is intrinsically better than another – but some appear to have a better chance of working in healthcare than others, and understanding the trade-offs that are involved in making decisions about how to organise health services is a central part of the debate about what kind of health services we want.

Appealing to intrinsic (not extrinsic) motivation

Some of the most robust research findings in psychology point to the need for organisational forms to appeal to the intrinsic rather than extrinsic motivations of staff within them (Pink, 2010). Instead of this, however, policy-makers seem to want to put in place performance management systems that are based on those working in health services chasing targets that seem to have little to do with good clinical practice, and to reorganise healthcare on market-based principles that seem to have little to do with encouraging the delivery of good care. Putting in place badly designed performance management systems seems to risk leading to what happened at Mid Staffordshire Hospital Trust, with targets being chased rather than patients being looked after. Market-based organisations, although they claim to offer greater choice, have cost the NHS billions over the last 20 years that could have been invested in better patient care instead.

Accountability, not markets

The present orthodoxy of healthcare organisation, that an increased use of markets is the way to make services more effective, responsive and efficient, is open to considerable doubt given the evidence presented in this book. While accepting the need to make health services more responsive to patients, it is necessary to understand that clinicians possess knowledge and experience that the vast majority of their patients lack. We need clinicians and patients to work together, with clinicians more aware of the service element of their roles, and patients respecting the knowledge and expertise of clinicians. Clinicians have to be held more accountable for the standard of their work through stronger peer review and closer regulation, but in a way that sets standards that allow buy-in from the professions rather than being imposed on them. In return, we need to accept that we have to adequately reward our clinicians, with nurses especially struggling with both their professional status alongside the still-dominant medics, and in terms of the still often poor financial rewards we afford them.

The QOF has shown that it is possible to set targets that clinicians accept as legitimate, and that they are prepared to work towards through partnerships across professional groupings and alongside managers. We need to extend the insights we can gain from considering the QOF to put in place specialty-based targets against which hospital-based interprofessional teams can be held to account, driving up standards and finding the sources of poor performance through a collaborative approach. There is scope for clinical teams to compete with one another towards greater achievement (as Muir Gray advocates on his website; see www.bvhc.co.uk and elsewhere), but this is competition based on raising clinical standards rather than the market-based, patient-chasing competition that the present healthcare reorganisation is based on.

Meaningful patient and public involvement

For meaningful PPI, deep and long-term relationships between health services and local people need to be established. If the NHS is to remain a public service, it needs to be made more accountable to those it serves. This can be a means of making sure health services become more responsive to local need at the individual level, by making sure that where things can be improved, or where things are going wrong, health services are being held to account and lessons learned. But improving PPI is also about allowing health services to become more locally specific – there is no reason why they have to be the same in both Clacton and Milton Keynes, where demographics and the health needs of local people are very different (Greener, 2008a). Health services need to be comprehensive in making sure treatment is available for everyone, and conform to national standards laid down in performance measures, but beyond that, it is surely part of the local democratic process that they be allowed to vary more to better serve local people, so long as this decision has been reached democratically.

Getting doctors and managers to work better together

Within our health services, finding ways of getting doctors and managers to work better together is another priority. Leadership and management development programmes need to support this aim, and encourage case-based understanding of the challenges the NHS and wider health system face from multiple perspectives. Educating clinicians about management (and/or leadership) does not provide generic answers to any problem – healthcare management, and indeed clinical practice, are inherently contextual and dependent on available resources and the cultures of those working in healthcare organisations. Successful healthcare management is about putting in place multiprofessional partnerships to reach agreed goals rather than trying to promote increased responsiveness through competition and fragmentation.

Improving healthcare management and leadership is a priority. In recent years, the NHS has been much exercised by ideas around leadership and governance, but has often struggled to say exactly what either of those things means or entails exactly. Part of the problem arises from the highly politicised environment that managers inhabit, which often prevents them leading or managing effectively since their political masters and mistresses often regard their role as to lead and manage even where they lack the requisite skills to do so (Blackler, 2006). Indeed, it is often the case that reorganisations derail promising local initiatives designed to both improve care and reduce waste in the system (Erskine et al, 2013). Training and consultancy courses and opportunities abound, the advertising of which suggests that those working in healthcare can dramatically improve both their own, and their organisational, effectiveness, if only they manage or lead better. But much of this training appears to ignore the research-based evidence considered in Chapter Six. Until leadership and management development/training programmes take greater account of the specific NHS context, they will surely fall short of the goal of improving healthcare. To get doctors and managers working better together, management development needs to help those responsible for running the NHS understand the institution within which they work, to explore differences in understandings about research between doctors and managers in a way that engages with both, and that leads to better mutual understanding through the use of case-based materials that reflect the challenges that they face together.

The answers don't lie in reorganisations

At the policy level, we desperately need our politicians to acknowledge that the large-scale, system-based reorganisation of health services is unlikely to be successful. In the early 1990s the first internal market attempted a 'big bang' reform, but policy-makers appeared to believe that the potential consequences of allowing a market, even at a highly managed level, to operate in the NHS were too risky. As a result, there was relatively little competition between providers, and the purchasing of care was rather more about continuity with the 1980s than with radical experimentation. In the 2000s, Labour extended the market to include greater private and not-for-profit provision. The results of Labour's reorganisation are seen by some researchers, especially those who have used particular quality measures, as demonstrating that competition can improve health services. However, the sheer volume of change during the 2000s, and the lack of relationship between different health service quality measures, makes it almost impossible to demonstrate or attribute any kind of simple causality. Equally, it seems puzzling that health economists advocating competition have not produced cost/benefit analyses of its introduction – even in clinical areas where improvements have been claimed. Could the significant expenditure on reorganisation not have been better used to employ more nurses and doctors, or invest in improved infrastructure?

The central problem with expecting large-scale, system-based reorganisation to improve health services is that it overlooks that healthcare is fundamentally about relationships between clinicians and patients as well as others, including managers. If those relationships can be better understood, aligned and improved, then healthcare will benefit.

Perhaps it is time that policy-makers were required, before they engage in significant organisational reform of any public service, to demonstrate that there is an evidence-based case for their proposals. This case might include a cost-benefit analysis of the proposed changes (as required with major infrastructure projects, and in which case, it is hard to see how virtually any reorganisation in the history of the NHS would have gone ahead), or by demonstrating that pilots of the proposals have been independently evaluated as having worked well before they are rolled out to the rest of the country. The present situation, where billions and billions have been spent on healthcare reorganisation, but to remarkably little effect, is not only a waste of money, but is also demoralising to hard-working staff, and risks care discontinuities for those the NHS is meant to be serving – its patients.

The logic of care

Much of what appears above is a plea for policy-makers to reconsider what our health service is for, and only then to think about how it should be organised. The answers do not lie in radical reorganisations, be they based on markets, or hierarchies, or anything else. Organisational forms can never improve care in themselves because they are only there to either support or frustrate those who are doing the caring. Surely we should start with care – the reason why we have health services – and work back from there?

The logic of care, as Mol (2008) makes clear, is based on a long-term, relatively open-ended partnership between clinicians and patients, requiring multidisciplinary teams, huge amounts of patience, and the will on both sides to try and make things better. Care is not about the fragmentation, time-limited, contractual and consumerist model that the mis-use of market mechanisms leads to. Care appeals to the intrinsic motivation of clinicians in reminding them why they trained as healthcare professionals and patients as a means of being well, rather than to extrinsic gains based on market relationships. If we start basing our health services on providing the best possible care, then we can go a long way in reminding ourselves of what they are for. We would argue that the principles outlined above go a considerable way towards supporting the logic of care, and so provide a strong basis for rethinking the way we organise our health services to these ends.

To conclude, we have pointed to alternative principles that seem to us to have a far better chance of succeeding in improving our health services than the essentially ideological market-based reorganisations that dominate thinking and the political discourse at present. Healthcare is too important (and too expensive!) to be based on ideas that have cost (and wasted) billions of pounds since their introduction in the 1990s, while achieving little of tangible benefit to justify the outlay. Perhaps the time has come for policy-makers to stop searching for silver bullet solutions to reforming healthcare, and instead allow those with the requisite skills and expertise to get on with the hard and messy business of healthcare improvement based on adhering to a set of principles that have a much better chance of succeeding.

References

Abbott, A. (1988) *The system of professions: An essay on the division of expert labor*, Chicago, IL: University of Chicago Press.

Abelson, J., Forest, P.-G., Eyles, J., Caseberr, A. and Mackean, G. (2004) 'Will it make a difference if I show up and share? A citizens' perspective on improving public involvement processes for health system decision-making', *Journal of Health Services Research & Policy*, vol 9, pp 205-12.

Alford, R. (1975) *Health care politics*, Chicago, IL: Univerity of Chicago Press.

Allen, D. (1995) 'Doctors in management or the revenge of the conquered: The role of management development for doctors', *Journal of Management in Medicine*, vol 9, pp 44-50.

Allen, P. and Jones, L. (2011) 'Diversity of health care providers', in N. Mays, A. Dixon and L. Jones (eds) *Understanding New Labour's market reforms of the English NHS*, London: The King's Fund, pp 16-29.

Allsop, J. and Jones, K. (2008) 'Withering the citizen, managing the consumer: Complaints in healthcare settings', *Social Policy and Society*, vol 7, pp 233-43.

Alshamsan, R., Millett, C., Majeed, A. and Khunti, K. (2010) 'Has pay for performance improved the management of diabetes in the United Kingdom?', *Primary Care Diabetes*, vol 4, pp 73-8.

Anders, E.A. (2009) *Development of professional expertise: Towards measurement of expert performance and design of optimal learning environments*, Cambridge: Cambridge University Press.

Andrews, R. and Martin, S. (2010) 'Regional variations in public service outcomes: The impact of policy divergence in England, Scotland and Wales', *Regional Studies*, vol 44, pp 919-34.

Appleby, J. and Dixon, J. (2004) 'Patient choice in the NHS: Having choice may not improve health outcomes', *British Medical Journal*, vol 329, no 7457, pp 61-2.

Archer, M. (1995) *Realist social theory: The morphogenetic approach*, Cambridge: Cambridge University Press.

Asenova, D. and Beck, M. (2003) 'The UK financial sector and risk management in PFI projects: A survey', *Public Money & Management*, vol 23, pp 195-202.

Asenova, D. and Beck, M. (2010) 'Crucial silences: When accountability met PFI and finance capital', *Critical Perspectives on Accounting*, vol 21, pp 1-13.

Audit Commision (1995) *The doctors' tale: The work of hospital doctors in England and Wales*, London: HMSO.

Audit Commission (1996) *What the doctor ordered*, London: Audit Commission.

Baggott, R. (1995) 'Controlling health professionals: The future of work and organization in the NHS', *Public Money & Management*, vol 15, pp 63-4.

Baggott, R. (1997) 'Evaluating health care reform: the case of the NHS internal market', *Public Administration*, vol 75, pp 283-306.

Baggott, R. (2005) 'A funny thing happened on the way to the forum? Reforming patient and public involvement in the NHS in England', *Public Administration*, vol 83, pp 533-51.

Baggott, R. (2006) *Understanding health policy*, Bristol: Policy Press.

Barber, M. (2007) *Instruction to deliver: Tony Blair, the public services and the challenge of achieving targets*, London: Portico's Publishing.

Barnes, M., Newman, J., Knops, A. and Sullivan, H. (2003) 'Constituting "the public" in public participation', *Public Administration*, vol 81, pp 379-99.

Baxter, K., Glendinning, C. and Greener, I. (2011) 'The implications of personal budgets for the home care market', *Public Money & Management*, vol 31, no 2, pp 91-8.

Bennett, C. and Ferlie, E. (1996) 'Contracting in theory and in practice: some evidence from the NHS', *Public Administration*, vol 74, pp 49-66.

Berwick, D. (2013) *A promise to learn – a commitment to act: Improve the safety of patients in England*, London: National Advisory Group on the Safety of Patients in England.

Bevan G. (2011) 'Regulation and system management', in N. Mays, A. Dixon and A. Jones (eds) *Understanding New Labour's market reforms of the English NHS*, London: The King's Fund, pp 89-111.

Bevan, G. and Hood, C. (2006a) 'Health policy: Have targets improved performance in the English NHS?', *British Medical Journal*, vol 332, no 7538, pp 419-22.

Bevan, G. and Hood, C. (2006b) 'What's measured is what matters: Targets and gaming in the English public health care system', *Public Administration*, vol 84, pp 517-38.

Bevan, G. and Skellern, M. (2011) 'Does competition between hospitals improve clinical quality? A review of evidence from two eras of competition in the English NHS', *British Medical Journal*, vol 343, pp 1-7.

Birchall, J. (2003) 'Mutualism and the governance of foundation trusts', Paper presented at the Centre for Healthcare Management Conference, Manchester, 13 June.

Black, N. and Thompson, E. (1993) 'Obstacles to medical audit: British doctors speak', *Social Science & Medicine*, vol 36, pp 849-56.

Blackler, F. (2006) 'Chief executives and the modernization of the English National Health Service', *Leadership*, vol 2, no 1, pp 5-30.

Blackman, T., Elliott, E., Greene, A., Harrington, B., Hunter, D.J., Marks, L., McKee, L. and Williams, G.H. (2006) 'Performance assessment and wicked problems: the case of health inequalities', *Public Policy and Administration*, vol 21, no 2, pp 66-80.

Blackman, T., Hunter, D.J., Marks, L., Harrington, B., Elliott, E., Williams, G., Green, A. and McKee, L. (2010) 'Wicked comparisons: reflections on cross-national research about health inequalities in the UK', *Evaluation*, vol 16, no 1, pp 43-57.

Blackman, T., Elliott, E., Greene, A., Harrington, B.E., Hunter, D.J., Marks, L., McKee, L., Smith, K.E. and Williams, G.H. (2009) 'Tackling health inequalities in post-devolution Britain: Do targets matter?', *Public Administration*, vol 87, no 4, pp 762-79.

Bloomfield, B. (1991) 'The role of information systems in the NHS: Action at a distance and the fetish of calculation', *Social Studies of Science*, vol 21, pp 701-34.

Boland, T. and Silbergh, D. (1996) 'Managing for quality: the impact of quality management initiatives on administrative structure and resource management processes in public-sector organizations', *International Review of Administrative Sciences*, vol 62, pp 351-67.

Bolzan, N. and Gale, F. (2002) 'The citizenship of excluded groups: Challenging the consumerist agenda', *Social Policy & Administration*, vol 36, pp 363-75.

Bolzan, N., Smith, M., Mears, J. and Ansiewicz, R. (2001) 'Creating identities: Mental health consumer to citizen?', *Journal of Social Work*, vol 1, pp 317-28.

Boyett, I. and Finlay, D. (1995) 'The quasi-market, the entrepreneur and the effectiveness of the NHS business manager', *Public Administration*, vol 73, pp 393-411.

Bradshaw, P.L. (2008) 'Service user involvement in the NHS in England: genuine user participation or a dogma-driven folly?', *Journal of Nursing Management*, vol 16, pp 673-81.

Braithwaite, J. and Westbrook, M. (2004) 'A survey of staff attitudes and comparative managerial and non-managerial views in a clinical directorate', *Health Services Management Research*, vol 17, pp 141-66.

Brearley, S. (1996) 'Seriously deficient professional performance', *British Medical Journal*, vol 312, pp 1180-1.

Broadbent, J. (1998) 'Practice nurses and the effects of the new general practitioner contract in the British NHS: The advent of a professional project?', *Social Science & Medicine*, vol 47, pp 497-506.

Brown, A. (1992) 'Managing change in the NHS: The resource management initiative', *Leadership & Organization Development Journal*, vol 13, pp 13-17.

Bryan, S., Gill, P., Greenfield, S., Gutridge, K. and Marshall, T. (2006) 'The myth of agency and patient choice in health care? The case of drug treatments to prevent coronary disease', *Social Science & Medicine*, vol 63, pp 2698-701.

Buchanan, D., Jordon, S., Perston, D. and Smith, A. (1997) 'Doctor in the process: The engagement of clinical directors in hospital management', *Journal of Management in Medicine*, vol 11, pp 132-56.

Butler, T. and Roland, M. (1998) 'How will primary care groups work?', *British Medical Journal*, vol 316, p 214.

Buxton, M. and Packwood, T. (1991) *Hospitals in transition: The resource management initiative*, Buckingham: Open University Press.

Callaghan, G. and Wistow, G. (2006a) 'Governance and public involvement in the British National Health Service: Understanding difficulties and developments', *Social Science & Medicine*, vol 63, pp 2289-300.

Callaghan, G. and Wistow, G. (2006b) 'Publics, patients, citizens, consumers? Power and decision making in primary health care', *Public Administration*, vol 84, pp 583-601.

Campbell, D. (2012) 'Hospital trusts offered £1.5bn emergency fund to pay PFI bill', *The Guardian*, 13 February.

Carr, S.M., Lhussier, M., Reynolds, Hunter, J.D. and Hannaway, C. (2009) 'Leadership for health improvement – implementation and evaluation', *Journal of Health Organization and Management*, vol 23, pp 200-15.

Chang, L., Lin, S. and Northcott, D. (2002) 'The NHS performance assessment framework: A "balanced scorecard" approach?', *Journal of Management in Medicine*, vol 16, pp 345-58.

CHE (Centre for Health Economics) (2012) *Hospital quality competition under fixed prices*, CHE Research Paper 80, York: University of York.

Checkland, K., McDonald, R. and Harrison, S. (2007) 'Ticking boxes and changing the social world: Data collection and the new UK general practice contract', *Social Policy & Administration*, vol 41, pp 693-710.

Checkland, K., Harrison, S., McDonald, R., Grant, S., Campbell, S. and Guthrie, B. (2008) 'Biomedicine, holism and general medical practice: responses to the 2004 general practitioner contract', *Sociology of Health & Illness*, vol 30, pp 788-803.

CHI (Commission for Health Improvement) (2001) *A guide for clinical governance reviews in NHS trusts*, London: CHI.

CHI (2003) *What CHI has found in ambulance services*, London: HSMO.

CHI (2004) *What CHI has found in acute services*, London: HMSO.

Clarke, J. (2004) *Changing welfare, changing welfare states*, London: Sage Publications.

Clarke, J. (2005) 'New Labour's citizens: activated, empowered, responsibilized, abandoned?', *Critical Social Policy*, vol 25, pp 447-63.

Clarke, J., Newman, J., Smith, N., Vidler, E. and Westmarland, L. (2007) *Creating citizen-consumers: Changing publics and changing public services*, London: Paul Chapman Publishing.

Clwyd, A. and Hart, P. (2013) *A review of the NHS hospitals complaints system: Putting patients back in the picture*, London: Department of Health.

Coleman, A., Checkland, K. and Harrison, S. (2009) 'Still puzzling: Patient and public involvement in commissioning', *Journal of Integrated Care*, vol 17, pp 23-30.

Colvin, G. (2008) *Talent is overrated. What really separates world-class performers from everyone else*, London: Nicholas Brealey Publishing Ltd.

Connolly, S., Bevan, G. and Mays, N. (2010) *Funding and performance of healthcare systems in the four countries of the UK before and after devolution*, London: Nuffield Trust.

Cooper, Z., Gibbons, S., Jones, S. and McGuire, A. (2011) 'Does hospital competition save lives? Evidence from the English NHS Patient Choice reforms', *Economic Journal*, vol 121, F229-F260.

Coulter, A., le Maistre, N. and Henderson, L. (2005) *Patients' experience of choosing where to undergo surgical treatment: Evaluation of the London Patient Choice Scheme*, Oxford: Picker Institute Europe.

Currie, G. (1996) 'Contested terrain: The incomplete closure of managerialism in the health service', *Personnel Review*, vol 25, pp 8-22.

Currie, G. (1998) 'Stakeholders' views of management development as a cultural change process in the health service', *Journal of Public Sector Management*, vol 11, pp 43-61.

Currie, G. (1999) 'Resistance around a management development programme: Negotiated order in a hospital trust', *Management Learning*, vol 30, pp 43-61.

Currie, G., Finn. R. and Martin, G. (2009) 'Professional competition and modernizing the clinical workforce in the NHS', *Work, Employment & Society*, vol 23, pp 267-84.

Currie, G. and Suhomlinova, O. (2006) 'The impact of international forces upon knowledge sharing in the UK NHS: The triumph of professional power and the inconsistency of policy', *Public Administration*, vol 84, no 1, pp 1-30

Curtice, J. and Heath, O. (2012) 'Does choice deliver? Public satisfaction with the health service', *Political Studies*, vol 60, pp 484-503.

Davies, H.T.O. and Mannion, R. (2013) 'Will prescriptions for cultural change improve the NHS?', *British Medical Journal*, vol 346, f1305.

Davies, H.T.O., Hodges, C. and Rundall, T.G. (2003) 'Views of doctors and managers on the doctor–manager relationship in the NHS', *British Medical Journal*, vol 326, no 7390, pp 626-8.

Davies, H.T.O., Nutley, S. and Smith, P.C. (1999) 'What works? The role of evidence in public sector policy and practice', *Public Money & Management*, vol 19, pp 3-5.

Davies, H.T.O., Nutley, S. and Smith, P.C. (2000) *What works? Evidence-based policy and practice in public services*, Bristol: Policy Press.

Davies, S. (2006) 'Health services management education: why and what?', *Journal of Health Organization and Management*, vol 20, pp 325-34.

Day, M. (2007) 'The rise of the doctor-manager', *British Medical Journal*, vol 335, pp 230-1.

Day, P. and Klein, R. (1991) 'Britain's health care experiment', *Health Affairs*, vol 10, pp 40-59.

Degeling, P., Kennedy, A. and Hill, M. (2001) 'Mediating the cultural boundaries between medicine, nursing and management – the central challenge of hospital reform', *Health Services Management Research*, vol 14, pp 36-48.

Degeling, P., Maxwell, S., Iedema, R. and Hunter, D. (2004) 'Making clinical governance work', *British Medical Journal*, vol 329, 18 September, pp 679-81.

Degeling, P., Maxwell, S., Kennedy, J. and Coyle, B. (2003) 'Medicine, management, and modernisation: a "danse macabre"?', *British Medical Journal*, vol 326, no 7390, pp 649-52.

Degeling, P., Zhang, K., Coyle, B., Xu, L., Meng, Q., Qu, J. and Hill, M. (2006) 'Clinicians and the governance of hospitals: A cross-cultural perspective on relations between profession and management', *Social Science & Medicine*, vol 63, pp 757-75.

Dent, M. and Haslam, C. (2006) 'Delivering patient choice in English acute hospital trusts', *Accounting Forum*, vol 30, pp 359-76.

DH (Department of Health) (1999) 'Clinical governance: in the new NHS', *Health Service Circular*, London: DH.

DH (2001a) *The expert patient: A new approach to chronic disease management for the 21st century*, London: DH.

DH (2001b) *Extending choice for patients*, London: DH.

DH (2001c) *NHS performance ratings: Acute trusts 2000/2001*, London: DH.

DH (2001d) *Shifting the balance of power within the NHS: Securing delivery*, London: The Stationery Office.

DH (2002) *Reforming NHS financial flows. Introducing payment by results*, London: DH.

DH (2005) *A short guide to NHS foundation trusts*, London: DH Publications.

DH (2006) *Patient choice becomes a reality across the NHS*, London: DH.

DH (2013) *What is Healthwatch?*, London: DH (http://healthandcare. dh.gov.uk/what-is-healthwatch).

DHSS (Department of Health and Social Security) (1983) *NHS management inquiry*, London: HMSO.

Dickinson, H. and Glasby, J. (2010) 'Why partnership working doesn't work', *Public Management Review*, vol 12, no 6, pp 811-26.

Dixon, A. and Jones, L. (2011) 'Local implementation of New Labour's market reforms', in N. Mays, A. Dixon and L. Jones (eds) *Understanding New Labour's market reforms of the English NHS*, London: The King's Fund, pp 112-23.

Dixon, A. and Mays, N. (2011) 'Lessons for future health care reforms in England', in N. Mays, A. Dixon and L. Jones (eds) *Understanding New Labour's market reforms of the English NHS*, London: The King's Fund, pp 143-60.

Dixon, A. and Robertson, R. (2011) 'Patient choice of hospital', in N. Mays, A. Dixon and L. Jones (eds) *Understanding New Labour's market reforms of the English NHS*, London: The King's Fund, pp 52-65.

Dixon, A., Storey, J. and Alvarez Rosete, A. (2010a) 'Accountability of foundation trusts in the English NHS: views of directors and governors', *Journal of Health Services Research & Policy*, vol 15, pp 82-9.

Dixon, A., Appleby, J., Robertson, R., Burge, P., Devlin, N. and Magee, H. (2010b) *Patient Choice – How patients choose and how providers respond*, London: The King's Fund.

Dixon, J. (2004) 'Payment by results – new financial flows in the NHS: The risks are large but may be worth while because of potential gains', *British Medical Journal*, vol 328, no 7446, pp 969-70.

Dixon, S. (2009) *Report on the National Patient Choice Survey – December 2008 England*, London: Department of Health.

Dixon, S. and Wright, N. (2008) *Report on the National Patient Choice Survey – July 2006*, London: Department of Health.

Donaldson, L.J. (1994) 'Doctors with problems in an NHS workforce', *British Medical Journal*, vol 308, pp 1277-82.

Donaldson, L.J. (2000) *An organisation with a memory – Report of an expert group on learning from adverse events in the NHS*, London: The Stationery Office.

Drucker, P. (1955) *The practice of management*, London: Heinemann.

Easington PCT (Primary Care Trust) (2006) *Choosing your hospital*, Peterlee: Easington PCT.

Edwards, A. and Langley, A. (2007) 'Understanding how general practices addressed the Quality and Outcomes Framework of the 2003 General Medical Services contract in the UK: a qualitative study of the effects on quality and team working of different approaches used', *Quality in Primary Care*, vol 15, pp 265-75.

Enthoven, A.C. (1985) *Reflections on the management of the National Health Service: An American looks at incentives to efficiency in health service management in the UK*, London: Nuffield Provincial Hospitals Trust.

Enthoven, A.C. (2000) 'In pursuit of an improving National Health Service', *Health Affairs*, vol 19, pp 102-19.

Erskine, J., Hunter, D., Small, A., Hicks, C., McGovern, T., Lugsden, E., Whitty, P., Steen, N. and Eccles, M. (2013) 'The role of leaders in enabling transformational change in healthcare organisations: Lessons from the North East Transformation System', *Health Services Management Research*, vol 26, no 1, pp 29-37.

Exworthy, M. and Halford, S. (1998) *Professionalism and the new managerialism in the public sector*, Buckingham: Open University Press.

Exworthy, M. and Peckham, S. (2006) 'Access, choice and travel: Implications for health policy', *Social Policy & Administration*, vol 40, June, pp 267-87.

Exworthy, M., Frosini, F. and Jones, L. (2011) 'Are NHS foundation trusts able and willing to exercise autonomy? "You can take a horse to water..."', *Journal of Health Services Research & Policy*, vol 16, pp 232-7.

Exworthy, M., Wilkinson, E.K., McColl, A., Moore, M., Roderick, P., Smith, H. and Gabbay, J. (2003) 'The role of performance indicators in changing the autonomy of the general practice profession in the UK', *Social Science & Medicine*, vol 56, pp 1493-504.

Farrar, S., Deokhee, Y. and Boyle, S. (2011) 'Payment by results', in N. Mays, A. Dixon and L. Jones (eds) *Understanding New Labour's market reforms of the English NHS*, London: The King's Fund, pp 66-77.

Fitzgerald, L. (1994) 'Moving clinicians into management: A professional challenge or threat?', *Journal of Management in Medicine*, vol 8, pp 32-44.

Fleetcroft, R. and Cookson, R. (2006) 'Do the incentive payments in the new NHS contract for primary care reflect likely population health gains?', *Journal of Health Services Research & Policy*, vol 11, pp 27-31.

Forbes, T., Hallier, J. and Kelly, L. (2004) 'Doctors as managers: investors and reluctants in a dual role', *Health Services Management Research*, vol 17, pp 167-76.

Ford, S., Schofield, T. and Hope, T. (2006) 'Observing decision-making in the general practice consultation: who makes which decisions?', *Health Expectations*, vol 9, pp 130-7.

Forster, R. and Gabe, J. (2008) 'Voice or choice? Patient and public involvement in the National Health Service in England under New Labour', *International Journal of Health Services*, vol 38, pp 333-56.

Fotaki, M., Boyd, A., Smith, L., McDonald, R., Roland, M., Sheaff, R., Edwards, A. and Elwyn, G. (2005) *Patient choice and the organization and delivery of health services: Scoping review*, London: National Coordinating Centre for the Service Delivery and Organisation.

Francis, R. (2010) *Independent inquiry into care provided by Mid Staffordshire NHS Foundation Trust January 2005-March 2009*, Chaired by Robert Francis, HC 375-1, London: The Stationery Office.

Francis, R. (2013) *Report of the Mid Staffordshire Foundation NHS Trust Public Inquiry Volumes 1-3*, HC-898-I-III, London: The Stationery Office.

Freedman, D.B. (2002) 'Clinical governance-bridging management and clinical approaches to quality in the UK', *Clinica Chimica Acta*, vol 319, pp 133-41.

Frey, B.S. and Osterloh, M. (2002) *Successful management by motivation: Balancing intrinsic and extrinsic incentives*, Berlin, Heidelberg and New York: Springer.

Frey. B.S. and Osterloh, M. (2012) 'Stop tying pay to performance: The evidence is overwhelming: It doesn't work', *Harvard Business Review*, January-February (http://hbr.org/2012/01/tackling-business-problems).

Gaynor, M., Moreno-Serra, R. and Propper, C. (2010) *Death by market power: Reform, competition and patient outcomes in the English National Health Service*, CMPO University of Bristol Working Paper 10/242, Bristol: Centre for Market and Public Organisation, University of Bristol.

Gaynor, M., Moreno-Serra, R. and Propper, C. (2012) 'Can competition improve outcomes in UK health care? Lessons from the past two decades', *Journal of Health Services Research & Policy*, vol 17, pp 49-54.

Giaimo, S. (1995) 'Health care reform in Britain and Germany: Recasting the political bargain with the medical profession', *Governance*, vol 8, pp 354-79.

Giddens, A. (2002) *What now for New Labour?*, Cambridge: Polity Press.

Glasby, J., Dickinson, H. and Miller, R. (2011) 'Partnership working in England – Where we are now and where we've come from', *International Journal of Integrated Care*, vol 11, March, pp 1-8.

Glennerster, H., Matsaganis, M., Owens, P. and Hancock, S. (1994) *Implementing GP fundholding:Wild card or winning hand?*, Buckingham: Open University Press.

Goddard, M., Mannion, R. and Smith, P.C. (1999) 'Assessing the performance of NHS hospital trusts: the role of "hard" and "soft" information', *Health Policy*, vol 48, pp 119-34.

Goodwin, N. (1998) 'GP fundholding', in J. Le Grand, N. Mays and J. Mulligan (eds) *Learning from the NHS internal market – A review of the evidence*, London: The King's Fund.

Green, J. (2006) 'Patient choice: A sociological perspective', *Journal of Health Services Research & Policy*, vol 11, pp 131-2.

Greener, I. (2001) '"The ghost of health services past" revisited: Comparing British health policy of the 1950s with the 1980s and 1990s', *International Journal of Health Services*, vol 31, pp 635-46.

Greener, I. (2002) 'Understanding NHS reform: The policy-transfer, social learning, and path-dependency perspectives', *Governance*, vol 15, pp 161-84.

Greener, I. (2003) 'Patient choice in the NHS: the view from economic sociology', *Social Theory & Health*, vol 1, pp 72-89.

Greener, I. (2004a) 'The drama of health management', in M. Learmonth and N. Harding (eds) *Unmaking health*, New York: Nova Science, pp 143-55.

Greener, I. (2004b) 'The three moments of New Labour's health policy discourse', *Policy & Politics*, vol 32, pp 303-16.

Greener, I. (2005) 'Health management as strategic behaviour: Managing medics and performance in the NHS', *Public Management Review*, vol 7, pp 95-110.

Greener, I. (2008a) *Healthcare in the UK: Understanding continuity and change*, Bristol: Policy Press.

Greener, I. (2008b) 'Markets in the public sector: when do they work, and what do we do when they don't?', *Policy & Politics*, vol 36, pp 93-108.

Greener, I. (2008c) 'Decision making in a time of significant reform: Managing in the NHS', *Administration & Society*, vol 40, no 4, pp 194-210.

Greener, I. (2009) 'Towards a history of choice in UK health policy', *Sociology of Health and Illness*, vol 31, pp 309-42.

Greener, I. (2012) 'Unpacking the evidence on competition and outcomes in the NHS in England', *Journal of Health Services Research & Policy*, vol 7, pp 193-5.

Greener, I. and Mannion, R. (2006) 'Does practice-based commissioning avoid the problems of fundholding?', *British Medical Journal*, vol 333, 2 December, pp 1168-70.

Greener, I and Mannion, R. (2009a) 'Patient choice in the NHS: what is the effect of choice policies on patients and relationships in health economies?', *Public Money & Management*, vol 29, pp 95-100.

Greener, I. and Mannion, R. (2009b) 'A realistic evaluation of practice-based commissioning', *Policy & Politics*, vol 37, pp 57-73.

Greener, I. and Powell, M. (2009) 'The evolution of choice policies in UK housing, education and health policy', *Journal of Social Policy*, vol 38, pp 63-81.

Greer, S. and Trench, A. (2008) *Health and intergovernmental relations in the devolved United Kingdom*, London: Nuffield Trust.

Griseri, P. (2002) *Management knowledge: A critical view*, London: Palgrave.

Gunstone, C. (2007) 'QOF', *British Journal of General Practice*, September, p 748.

Ham, C. (1996) 'Managed markets in health care: the UK experiment', *Health Policy*, vol 35, pp 279-92.

Ham, C. (1999) 'Improving NHS performance: human behaviour and health policy', *British Medical Journal*, vol 319, pp 1490-2.

Ham, C. (2000) *The politics of NHS reform 1988-97: Metaphor or reality?*, London: The King's Fund.

Hamer, L. (2003) *Local government scrutiny for health: Using the new power to tackle health inequalities*, London: Health Development Agency.

Harrington, B.E., Smith, K.E., Hunter, D.J., Marks, L., Blackman, T.J., McKee, L., Greene, A., Elliott, E. and Williams, G.H. (2009) 'Health inequalities in England, Scotland, and Wales: stakeholders' accounts and policy compared', *Public Health*, vol 123, e24-e28.

Harrison, S. (1988) *Managing the National Health Service: Shifting the frontier?*, London: Chapman & Hall.

Harrison, S. (2002) 'New Labour, modernisation and the medical labour process', *Journal of Social Policy*, vol 31, pp 465-85.

Harrison, S. and Dowswell, G. (2002) 'Autonomy and bureaucratic accountability in primary care: what English general practitioners say', *Sociology of Health & Illness*, vol 24, pp 208-26.

Harrison, S. and Pollitt, C. (1994) *Controlling health professionals – The future of work and organisation in the NHS*, Buckingham: Open University Press.

Harrison, S. and Wistow, G. (1992) 'The purchaser/provider split in English health care: towards explicit rationing?', *Policy & Politics*, vol 20, pp 123-30.

Harrison, S., Hunter, D.J. and Pollitt, C. (1990) *The dynamics of British health policy*, London: Unwin Hyman.

Harrison, S., Hunter, D.J., Marnoch, G. and Pollitt, C. (1992) *Just managing: Power and culture in the NHS*, London: Macmillan.

Hart, C. (1994) *Behind the mask: Nurses, their unions and nursing policy*, London: Bailliere Tindall.

Headrick, L.A., Wilcock, P.M. and Batalden, P.B. (1998) 'Interprofessional working and continuing medical education', *British Medical Journal*, vol 316, pp 771-4.

Healthcare Commission (2009) *Investigation into Mid Staffordshire NHS Foundation Trust*, London: Healthcare Commission.

Heath, G. and Radcliffe, J. (2007) 'Performance measurement and the English Ambulance Service', *Public Money & Management*, vol 27, pp 223-8.

Hirschman, A. (1970) *Exit, voice and loyalty: Responses to decline in firms, organizations and states*, London: Harvard University Press.

HM Government (2010) *The Coalition: Our programme for government*, London: Cabinet Office.

Holman, D. and Hall, L. (1996) 'Competence in management development: Rites and wrongs', *British Journal of Management*, vol 7, pp 191-202.

Hood, C. (1991) 'A public management for all seasons?', *Public Administration*, vol 69, Spring, pp 3-19.

Hood, C. (2006) 'Gaming in Targetworld: The targets approach to managing British public services', *Public Administration Review*, vol 66, pp 515-21.

Horrocks, S. and Coast, J. (2007) 'Patient choice: an exploration of primary care dermatology patients' values and expectations of care', *Quality in Primary Care*, vol 15, pp 185-93.

House of Commons Health Committee (2009) *Commisioning, Fourth report of Session 2009-10, Volume 1*, London: House of Commons.

Hudson, B. (2012) 'Twenty years of health and social care joint working: a journey from Doctor Pangloss to Private Frazer?', *Journal of Integrated Care*, vol 20, no 2, pp 115-24.

Hudson, B. and Hardy, B. (2002) 'What is a successful "partnership" and how can it be measured?', in C. Glendinning, M. Powell and K. Rummery, *Partnerships, New Labour and the governance of welfare*, Bristol: Policy Press, pp 51-65.

Hudson, S. (2009) 'Is the QOF failing to motivate GPs or improve patient care? Evidence from an exploratory study', *Journal of Primary Care*, September, pp 1-5.

Hughes, D., Mullen, C. and Vincent-Jones, P. (2009) 'Choice vs voice? PPI policies and the re-positioning of the state in England and Wales', *Health Expectations*, vol 12, pp 237-50.

Hunter, D.J. (1996) 'The changing roles of health care personnel in health and health care management', *Social Science & Medicine*, vol 43, pp 799-808.

Hunter, D.J. (2003) 'Foundation hospitals: Back to the future', *Public Money & Management*, vol 23, pp 211-13.

Hunter, D.J. (2006) 'From tribalism to corporatism: the continuing managerial challenge to medical dominance', in D. Kelleher, J. Gabe and G. Williams (eds) *Challenging medicine*, Basingtoke: Routledge, pp 1-22.

Hunter, D.J. (2008) *The health debate*, Bristol: Policy Press.

Hunter, D.J. (2011) 'Change of government: one more big bang health care reform in England's National Health Service', *International Journal of Health Services*, vol 41, no 1, pp 159-74.

Hunter, D.J. (2013a) 'A response to Rudolf Klein: A battle may have been won but perhaps not the war', *Journal of Health Policy, Politics and Law*, vol 38, no 4, pp 869-75.

Hunter D.J. (2013b) 'Health inequality and govenance in Scotland since 2007', *Public Health*, vol 127, no 6, pp 3, 517.

Hunter, D.J. and Perkins, N. (2012) 'Partnership working in public health: The implications for governance of a systems approach', *Journal of Health Services Research & Policy*, vol 17, suppl 2, pp 45-52.

Iliffe, S. and Munro, J. (2000) 'New Labour and Britain's National Health Service: An overview of current reforms', *International Journal of Health Services*, vol 30, pp 309-34.

Iyengar, S. (2010) *The art of choosing*, London: Hachette Digital.

Jahrami, H., Marnoch, G. and Gray, A. (2009) 'Use of card sort methodology in the testing of a clinical leadership competencies model', *Health Services Management Research*, vol 22, pp 176-83.

Kennedy, I. (2001) *Learning from Bristol: The report of the public inquiry into children's heart surgery at the Bristol Royal Infirmary 1984-1995*, Cm 5207, London: The Stationery Office.

Keogh, B. (2013) *Review into the quality of care and treatment provided by 14 hospital trusts in England*, NHS England.

Kitchener, M. (1997) 'Quasi-market transformation: An institutionalist approach to change in UK hospitals', *Public Administration*, vol 76, pp 73-95.

Kitchener, M. (2000) 'The "bureaucratization" of professional roles: The case of clinical directors in UK hospitals', *Organization*, vol 7, pp 129-54.

Klein, R. (1979) 'Ideology, class and the National Health Service', *Journal of Health Politics, Policy and Law*, vol 4, pp 464-90.

Klein, R. (1990) 'The state and the profession: the politics of the double-bed', *British Medical Journal*, vol 301, no 3, October, pp 700-2.

Klein, R. (1995) 'Big bang health care reform: Does it work? The case of Britain's 1991 National Health Service reforms', *Milbank Quarterly*, vol 73, pp 299-337.

Klein, R. (1999) 'Editorials – Markets, politicians, and the NHS: Enthoven's analysis still illuminates the NHS', *British Medical Journal*, vol 319, pp 1383-4.

Klein, R. (2003) 'Governance for NHS foundation trusts: Mr Milburn's flawed model is a cacophony of accountabilities', *British Medical Journal*, vol 326, no 7382, pp 174-5.

Klein, R. (2006) *The new politics of the NHS: From creation to reinvention*, Abingdon: Radcliffe Publishing.

Klein, R. (2013) 'The twenty-year war over England's National Health Service: A report from the battlefield', *Journal of Health Politics, Policy and Law*, vol 38, no 4, pp 849-69.

Klein, R. and Maynard, A. (1998) 'On the way to Calvary: Ministers should realise the command and control model the white paper entails', *British Medical Journal*, vol 317, pp 5-10.

Laughlin, R. (1991) 'Can the information systems for the NHS internal market work?', *Public Money & Management*, vol 11, pp 37-41.

Laverty, A., Smith, P., Paper Utz, J., Mears, A., Wachter, R. and Millett, C. (2012) 'High-profile investigations into hospital safety problems in England did not prompt patients to switch providers', *Health Affairs*, vol 31, pp 593-601.

Lawson, N. (1991) *The view from No 11*, London: Corgi.

Le Grand, J. (1991) 'Quasi-markets and social policy', *The Economic Journal*, vol 101, pp 1256-67.

Le Grand, J. (2007) *The other invisible hand*, Woodstock: Princetown University Press.

Le Grand, J. (2011) 'Cameron's NHS reform is no health revolution', *Financial Times*, 19 January.

Le Grand, J., Mays, N. and Mulligan, J. (1998) *Learning from the NHS internal market*, London: The King's Fund.

Learmonth, M. and Harding, N. (2006) 'Evidence-based management: The very idea', *Public Administration*, vol 84, pp 245-66.

Learmonth, M., Martin, G.P. and Warwick, P. (2009) 'Ordinary and effective: the catch-22 in managing the public voice in health care?', *Health Expectations*, vol 12, pp 106-15.

Leese, B. (2007) 'New opportunities for nurses and other healthcare professionals? A review of the potential impact of the new GMS contract on the primary care workforce', *Journal of Health Organization and Management*, vol 20, pp 525-36.

Lempp, H. (1995) 'Has nursing lost its way? Nursing: no regrets', *British Medical Journal*, vol 311, pp 307-8.

Lewis, R.Q. (2005) 'NHS foundation trusts: The Healthcare Commission's review offers something for both proponents and detractors', *British Medical Journal*, vol 331, no 7508, pp 59-60.

Light, D.W. (1992) 'The radical experiment: Transforming Britain's National Health System to interlocking markets', *Journal of Public Health Policy*, vol 13 (Summer), pp 146-55.

Light, D.W. (1998) 'Is NHS purchasing serious? An American perspective', *British Medical Journal*, vol 316, pp 217-20.

Likierman, A. (1993) 'Performance indicators: 20 early lessons from managerial use', *Public Money & Management*, vol 13, pp 15-22.

Llewellyn, S. (2001) '"Two-way windows": Clinicians as medical managers', *Organization Studies*, vol 22, pp 593-623.

Lovett, J. and Curry, A. (2007) 'Quality improvement with the new general practitioner contract – myth or reality?', *Health Services Management Research*, vol 20, pp 121-33.

McCafferty, S., Williams. I., Hunter, D.J., Robinson, S., Donaldson, C. and Bate, A. (2012) 'Implementing world class commissioning competencies', *Journal of Health Services Research & Policy*, vol 17, suppl 1, pp 40-8.

McCartney, M. (2012) *The patient paradox: Why sexed up medicine is bad for your health*, London: Pinter and Martin Ltd.

McDonald, R., Checkland, K. and Harrison, S. (2009a) 'The new GP contract in English primary health care: an ethnographic study', *International Journal of Public Sector Management*, vol 22, pp 21-34.

McDonald, R., Harrison, S. and Checkland, K. (2008) 'Identity, contract and enterprise in a primary care setting: An English general practice case study', *Organization*, vol 15, pp 355-70.

McDonald, R., Campbell, S. and Lester, H. (2009b) 'Practice nurses and the effects of the new general practitioner contract in the English National Health Service: The extension of a professional project?', *Social Science & Medicine*, vol 68, pp 1206-12.

McDonald, R., Harrison, S., Checkland, K., Campbell, S.M. and Roland, M. (2007) 'Impact of financial incentives on clinical autonomy and internal motivation in primary care: ethnographic study', *British Medical Journal*, vol 334, p 1357.

McGucken, R.B. (1994) 'Medical directors of trusts should have clinical duties ... particularly in acute trusts', *British Medical Journal*, vol 308, pp 982-3.

McKee, M. (2004) 'Commentary: Not everything that counts can be counted; not everything that can be counted counts', *British Medical Journal*, vol 328, no 7432, p 153.

McLellan, A. (2012) 'A weak private sector is bad news for the NHS', *Health Service Journal*, 26 January.

Maisey, S., Steel, N., Marsh, R., Gillam, S., Fleetcroft, R. and Howe, A. (2008) 'Effects of payment for performance in primary care: qualitative interview study', *Journal of Health Services Research & Policy*, vol 13, pp 133-9.

Mannion, R., Davies, H. and Marshall, M. (2005) 'Impact of star performance ratings in English acute hospital trusts', *Journal of Health Services Research & Policy*, vol 10, no 1, pp 18-24.

Mannion, R., Goddard, M., Kuhn, M. and Bate, A. (2003) *Earned autonomy in the NHS: A report for the Department of Health*, London: Department of Health.

Marshall, M. and McLoughlin, V. (2010) 'How do patients use information on health providers?', *British Medical Journal*, vol 341, 25 November.

Marnoch, G., McKee, L. and Dinnie, N. (2000) 'Between organizations and institutions. Legitimacy and medical managers', *Public Administration*, vol 78, pp 967-87.

Martin, G.P. (2008a) 'Representativeness, legitimacy and power in public involvement in health service management', *Social Science & Medicine*, vol 67, pp 1757-65.

Martin, G.P. (2008b) '"Ordinary people only": knowledge, representativeness, and the publics of public participation in healthcare', *Sociology of Health & Illness*, vol 30, pp 35-54.

Martin, G.P. (2009) 'Public and user participation in public service delivery: Tensions in policy and practice', *Sociology Compass*, vol 3, pp 310-26.

Matka, E., Barnes, M. and Sullivan, H. (2002) 'Health Action Zones: "Creating alliances to achieve change"', *Policy Studies*, vol 23, pp 97-106.

Maynard, A. (1994) 'Can competition enhance efficiency in health care? Lessons from the reform of the UK National Health Service', *Social Science & Medicine*, vol 39, pp 1433-45.

Mays, N. (2011) 'Is there evidence that competition is healthcare is a good thing? No', *British Medical Journal*, vol 343, d4205.

Mays, N. and Dixon, A. (2011) 'Assessing and explaining the impact of New Labour's market reforms', in N. Mays, A. Dixon and L. Jones (eds) *Understanding New Labour's market reforms of the English NHS*, London: The King's Fund, pp 124-42.

Mays, N., Dixon, A. and Jones, A. (2011) 'Return to the market: objectives and evolution of New Labour's market reforms', in A. Dixon, N. Mays and L. Jones (eds) *Understanding New Labour's market reforms of the English NHS*, London: The King's Fund, pp 1-15. anuary.

Merrison, A. (1979) *Royal Commission on the National Health Service: Report*, London: HMSO.

Milburn, A. (2011) 'The NHS debacle sets us back a generation', *Telegraph*, 15 June.

Mitton, C, Smith, N., Peacock, S., Evoy, B. and Abelson, J. (2009) 'Public participation in health care priority setting: A scoping review', *Health Policy*, vol 91, pp 219-28.

Mol, A. (2008) *The logic of care: Health and problem of patient choice*, London: Routledge.

Monitor (2008) *NHS foundation trusts: Review and consolidated accounts 2007-08*, London: Monitor.

Montgomerie, T. (2012) 'The unnecessary and unpopular NHS Bill could cost the Conservative Party the next election. Cameron must kill it', ConservativeHome (http://conservativehome.blogs.com/thetorydiary/2012/02/the-unnecessary-and-unpopular-nhs-bill-could-cost-the-conservative-party-the-next-election-cameron-m.html).

Mueller, F., Harvey, C. and Howarth, C. (2003) 'The contestation of archetypes: Negotiating scripts in a UK hospital trust board', *Journal of Management Studies*, vol 40, pp 1971-95.

Muir Gray, J. (1996) *Evidence-based health care*, New York: Churchill Livingstone.

Naylor, C., Curry, C., Holder, H., Ross, S., Marshall, L. and Tait, E. (2013) *Clinical comissioning groups: Supporting improvement in general practice?*, London: The King's Fund and Nuffield Trusts.

NHS Future Forum (2011) *NHS Future Forum recommendations to government*, London: NHS Future Forum.

Nio Ong, B. and Schepers, R. (1998) 'Comparative perspectives on doctors in management in the UK and The Netherlands', *Journal of Management in Medicine*, vol 12, pp 378-90.

Nwabueze, U. (2001) 'The implementation of TQM for the NHS manager', *Total Quality Management*, vol 12, pp 657-75.

O'Connor, A., Bennett, C., Stacey, D., Barry, M., Col, N., Eden, K., Entwistle, V., Fiset, V., Holmes-Rovner, M., Khangura, S., Llewellyn-Thomas, H. and Rovner, D. (2009) 'Decision aids for people facing health treatment or screening decisions (Review)', *Cochrane Library*, pp 1-113.

O'Reilly, D., Steele, K., Patterson, C., Milsom, P. and Harte, P. (2006) 'Might how you look influence how well you are looked after? A study which demonstrates that GPs perceive socio-economic gradients in attractiveness', *Journal of Health Services Research & Policy*, vol 11, pp 231-4.

Office of Public Services Reform (2005) *Choice and voice in the reform of public services: Goverment response to the PASC report – Choice, voice and public services*, Cm 6630, London: The Stationery Office.

Oliver, K., Everett, M., Verma, A. and de Vocht, F. (2012) 'The human factor: Re-organisations in public health policy.' *Health Policy*, vol 106, no 1, pp 97-103.

Owen, J. and Phillips, K. (2000) 'Ignorance is not bliss – Doctors, management and development', *Journal of Management in Medicine*, vol 14, pp 119-29.

Packwood, T., Buxton, M. and Keen, J. (1990) 'Resource management in the National Health Service: a first case history', *Policy & Politics*, vol 18, pp 245-55.

Packwood, T., Kerrison, S. and Buxton, M. (1994) 'The implementation of medical audit', *Social Policy & Administration*, vol 28, pp 299-316.

Pawson, R. (2006) *Evidence-based policy: A realist perspective*, London: Sage Publications.

Pawson, R. (2013) *The science of evaluation: A realist manifesto*, London: Sage.

Pawson, R., Greenhaigh, T., Harvey, G. and Walshe, K. (2005) 'Realist review – a new method of systematic review for complex policy interventions', *Journal of Health Services Research & Policy*, vol 10, July, pp 21-34.

Peckham, S., Exworthy, M., Greener, I. and Powell, M. (2005) *Decentralisation as an organisational model in England*, London: National Coordinating Centre for the Service Delivery and Organisation.

Perkins, N., Smith, K., Hunter, D.J., Bambra, C. and Joyce, K. (2010) '"What counts is what works?" New Labour and partnerships in public health', *Policy & Politics*, vol 38, pp 101-17.

Petchey, R. (1993) 'NHS internal market 1991-2: towards a balance sheet', *British Medical Journal*, vol 306, pp 699-701.

Pickard, S. (1998) 'Citizenship and consumerism in health care: A critique of Citizen's Juries', *Social Policy & Administration*, vol 32, pp 226-44.

Pink, D. (2010) *Drive:The suprising truth about what motivates us*, London: Cannongate Books.

Plochg, T. and Klazringa, N. (2005) 'Talking towards excellence: a theoretical underpinning of the dialogue between doctors and managers', *Clinical Governance*, vol 10, pp 41-8.

Pollitt, C. (1985) 'Measuring performance: A new system for the National Health Service', *Policy & Politics*, vol 13, pp 1-15.

Pollitt, C. (1993) 'The struggle for wuality: the case of the National Health Service', *Policy & Politics*, vol 21, pp 161-70.

Pollitt, C., Harrison, S., Hunter, D.J. and Marnoch, G. (1991) 'General management in the NHS: The initial impact 1983-88', *Public Administration*, vol 69, Spring, pp 61-83.

Pollock, A., Macfarlane, A., Kirkwood, G., Majeed, A., Greener, I., Morelli, C., Boyle, S., Mellett, H., Godden, S., Price, D. and Brhlikova, P. (2011) 'No evidence that patient choice in the NHS saves lives', *Lancet*, vol 378, pp 2057-60.

Powell, J.E. (1966) *Medicine and politics*, London: Pitman Medical.

Powell, M. (1997) *Evaluating the National Health Service*, Buckingham: Open University Press.

Powell, M. (1998) 'New Labour and the "new" UK NHS', *Critical Public Health*, vol 8, pp 167-73.

Powell, M. (2011) 'If only policy makers would engage with our evidence, we'd get better policy', in J. Glasby (ed) *Evidence, policy and practice: Critical perspectives in health and social care*, Bristol: Policy Press, pp 11-31.

Propper, C. (1995) 'Agency and incentives in the NHS internal market', *Social Science & Medicine*, vol 40, pp 1683-90.

Propper, C. and Dixon, J. (2011) 'Competitoin between hospitals', in N. Mays, A. Dixon and L. Jones (eds) *Understanding New Labour's market reforms of the English NHS*, London: The King's Fund, pp 78-88.

Propper, C., Sutton, M., Whitnall, C. and Windmeijer, F. (2010) 'Incentives and targets in hospital care: Evidence from a natural experiment', *Journal of Public Economics*, vol 94, pp 318-35.

Ramesh, R. (2010) 'NHS spends millions on websites that fail patients, says government report', *The Guardian*, 4 August (www.guardian.co.uk/society/2010/aug/04/nhs-websites-failing-patients?INTCMP=SRCH).

Ramesh, R. (2012) 'Ailing NHS hospital trusts receive multimillion-pound bailout', *The Guardian*, 5 July.

Rawnsley, A. (2010) *The end of the party: The rise and fall of New Labour*, London: Penguin.

Reedy, P. and Learmonth, M. (2000) 'Nursing managers: transformed or deformed? A case study in the ideology of competency', *Journal of Management in Medicine*, vol 14, pp 153-65.

Reid, J. (2004) 'Managing new realities – integrating the care landscape', Speech given on 11 March.

Richards, P. (1998) 'Professional self respect: rights and responsibilities in the new NHS', *British Medical Journal*, vol 317, pp 1146-8.

Richards, S. (2010) *Whatever it takes: The real story of Gordon Brown and New Labour*, London: Fourth Estate.

Riordan, J.F. and Simpson, J. (1994) 'Getting started as a medical manager', *British Medical Journal*, vol 309, pp 1563-5.

Robertson, R., Dixon, A. and Le Grand, J. (2008) 'Patient choice in general practice: the implications of patient satisfaction surveys', *Journal of Health Services Research & Policy*, vol 13, pp 67-72.

Robinson, R. and Le Grand, J. (1994) *Evaluating the NHS reforms*, vol 1, London: King's Fund Institute.

Rogers, W. (2002) 'Evidence-based medicine in practice: limiting or facilitating patient choice?', *Health Expectations*, vol 5, pp 95-103.

Rossiter, A. and Williams, J. (2005) 'Choice systems in practice: case study in health', *Consumer Policy Review*, vol 15, no 3, pp 85-93.

Rozmovits, L., Rose, P. and Ziebland, S. (2004) 'In the absence of evidence, who chooses? A qualitative study of patients' needs after treatment for colorectal cancer', *Journal of Health Services Research & Policy*, vol 9, pp 159-64.

Russell, E. (1998) 'The ethics of attribution: The case of health care outcome indicators', *Social Science & Medicine*, vol 47, pp 1161-9.

Russell, V., Wyness, L., McAuliffe, E. and Fellenz, M. (2010) 'The social identity of hospital consultants as managers', *Journal of Health Organization and Management*, vol 24, pp 220-36.

Salter, B. (1999) 'Change in the governance of medicine: the politics of self-regulation', *Policy & Politics*, vol 27, pp 143-58.

Sandford, D. (2001) 'Is medicine rotten to the core?', *BBC News*, 5 November.

Schwartz, B. (2004) *The paradox of choice: Why less is more*, New York: HarperCollins.

Secretary of State for Health (1989) *Working for patients*, Cmnd 555, London: HMSO.

Secretary of State for Health (1996) *The NHS: A service with ambitions*, London: HMSO.

Secretary of State for Health (1997) *The new NHS: Modern, dependable*, Cm 3807, London: The Stationery Office.

Secretary of State for Health (2000) *The NHS plan: A plan for investment, a plan for reform*, Cmnd 4818-I, London: The Stationery Office.

Secretary of State for Health (2010) *Equity and excellence: Liberating the NHS*, Cm 7881, London: The Stationery Office.

Sheaff, R. (2009) 'Medicine and management in English primary care: A shifting balance of power?', *Journal of Social Policy*, vol 38, pp 627-47.

Sheldon, T. (1990) 'When it makes sense to mince your words', *Health Service Journal*, 16 August, p 121.

Sibbald, B. (2008) 'Who needs doctors in general practice?', *Quality in Primary Care*, vol 16, pp 73-4.

Smith, J., Walshe, K. and Hunter, D.J. (2001) 'The "redisorganisation" of the NHS: another reorganisation leaving unhappy managers can only worsen the service', *British Medical Journal*, vol 323, pp 1262-3.

Smith, K.E., Hunter, D.J., Blackman, T., Elliott, E., Greene, A., Harrington, B.E., Marks, L., McKee, L. and Williams, G.H. (2009) 'Divergence or convergence? Health inequalities and policy in a devolved Britain', *Critical Social Policy*, vol 29, no 2, pp 216-42.

Smith, R. (2003) 'What doctors and managers can learn from one another. A lot', *British Medical Journal*, vol 326, 22 March, pp 610-11.

Som, C. (2005) 'Nothing seems to have changed, nothing seems to be changing and perhaps nothing will change in the NHS: doctors' response to clinical governance', *Clinical Governance*, vol 18, pp 463-77.

Southon, G. and Braithwaite, J. (1998) 'The end of professionalism?', *Social Science & Medicine*, vol 46, pp 23-8.

Spurgeon, P., Hicks, C., Field, S. and Barwell, F. (2005) 'The new GMS contract: impact and implications for managing the changes', *Health Services Management Research*, vol 18, pp 75-85.

Steel, D. and Cyclus, J. (2012) 'United Kingdom (Scotland): Health system review', *Health Systems in Transition*, vol 14, no 9, European Observatory of Health Systems and Policies, World Health Organization.

Stevens, S. (2004) 'Reform strategies for the English NHS', *Health Affairs*, vol 23, no 3, pp 37-44.

Stevens, S. (2010) 'NHS reform is a risk worth taking', *Financial Times*, 15 July.

Stevens, S. (2011) 'Interview: Making sense of the NHS reforms', Health Policy Insight (www.healthpolicyinsight.com/?q=node/1072).

Stoker, G. (2006) *Why politics matters: Making democracy work*, London: Palgrave.

Storey, J. and Buchanan, D. (2008) 'Healthcare governance and organizational barriers to learning from mistakes', *Journal of Health Organization and Management*, vol 22, pp 642-51.

Street, A. (2000) 'Confident about efficiency measurement in the NHS?', *Health Care UK*, Spring, pp 47-52.

Taylor, R. (2013) *God bless the NHS: The truth behind the current crisis*, London: Faber and Faber.

Timmins, N. (1995a) *The five giants*, London: Fontana.

Timmins, N. (1995b) 'How three top managers nearly sank the reforms', *Health Service Journal*, 29 June, pp 11-13.

Timmins, N. (2012) *Never again?*, London: The King's Fund and Institute for Government.

Timmins, N. (2013) *The four UK health systems: Learning from each other*, London: The King's Fund

Tudor-Hart, J. (1971) 'The inverse care law', *Lancet*, pp 405-12.

Vaughan, C. and Higgs, R. (1995) 'Doctors and commitment', *British Medical Journal*, vol 311, pp 1654-5.

Verzulli, R., Jacobs, R. and Goddard, M. (2011) *Do hospitals respond to greater autonomy? Evidence from the English NHS*, Working Papers, York: Centre for Health Economics, University of York.

Wainwright, D. (1998) 'Disenchantment, ambivalence and the precautionary principle: The becalming of British health policy', *International Journal of Health Services*, vol 28, pp 407-26.

Walshe, K. (2003) 'Foundation hospitals: a new direction for NHS reform?', *Journal of the Royal Society of Medicine*, vol 96, pp 106-10.

Walshe, K. and Rundall, T.G. (2001) 'Evidence-based management: From theory to practice in health care', *The Milbank Quarterly*, vol 79, pp 429-57.

Wanless, D. (2002) *Securing our future health: Taking a long term view – Final report*, London: HM Treasury.

Warner, N. (2011) *A suitable case for treatment: The NHS and reform*, London: Grosvener House Publishing.

Weir, N., Kotecha, M. and Goel, K. (2007) 'Expanding choice options for older patients in relation to practice-based commissioning: a qualitative study of older patients in a small GP surgery', *Quality in Primary Care*, vol 15, pp 331-6.

West, P. (1998) 'Market – what market? A review of health authority purchasing in the NHS internal market', *Health Policy*, vol 44, pp 167-83.

Williams, I., Dickinson, H. and Robinson, S. (2009) 'Clinical microsystems and the NHS: A sustainable method for improvement', *Journal of Health Organization and Management*, vol 23, pp 119-32.

Wilson, D. (2011) 'Comparative analysis in public management: reflections on the experience of a major research programme', *Public Management Review*, vol 13, pp 293-308.

Wistow, G. (2001) 'Modernisation, the NHS Plan and healthy communities', *Journal of Management in Medicine*, vol 15, pp 334-51.

Index

Note: The following abbreviations have been used – *n* = note; *t* = table